THE ANTIOXIDANT REVOLUTION

- AN IDEA OF LONGEVITY -

PRINCE N. AGBEDANU, PhD

Book Design: Nonon Tech & Design

First Printing, 2020

ISBN: 978-1-959642-00-8

Table of Contents

PART I:

Introduction

O xidation—the chemical reactions involving Oxygen—impact the quality of life in various ways. For example, oxidation of proteins reduces the nutritional values of food. The oxidation process and its outcomes remain highly researched areas in food science and health [1]. Oxidised proteins and the end products of oxidation reactions play integral roles in human health. They irreversibly damage our cellular proteins and promote various diseases due to their potential mutagenic, carcinogenic, and neurotoxic activities in the body [2]. However, this book presents premises that outline the implications of oxidation on life and how these free radicals can be stabilised and neutralised with antioxidants to improve the quality of life.

Therefore, the objective of this book is to provide a comprehensive review of health challenges related to oxidation, mechanisms of free radicals, factors promoting free radical activities in food and the human body. Additionally, we propose practical methods for decimating free radicals to reduce their impact on your DNA with an aim to improve the healthspan and lifespan using antioxidants. These and more will be discussed extensively in subsequent chapters.

CHAPTER ONE

The Process of Oxidation in Nutrition

O xidation is defined as a chemical reaction that occurs in the presence of Oxygen [1]. It is responsible for the declining quality of life and food products, including changes in flavour and colouration [3]. The oxidation process in the body damages your cell membranes and other complex body parts, including your DNA, cellular proteins, and lipids (figure 1) [4]. When Oxygen is metabolised, it produces unstable molecules called 'free radicals,' which capture electrons from other molecules of proteins, DNA, and lipids, thereby causing damage to your cells, tissues, and organs.

The body requires a small number of free radicals to maintain optimal function. However, an excess of free radicals causes irreversible damage to cellular molecules, contributing to several diseases, including heart failure, liver failure, various cancers, and degenerative diseases such as osteoporosis, Alzheimer's disease, and

Parkinson's [5, 6]. Oxidation can be exacerbated by stress, pollution, tobacco smoking, alcohol, sunlight, and other environmental and lifestyle factors.

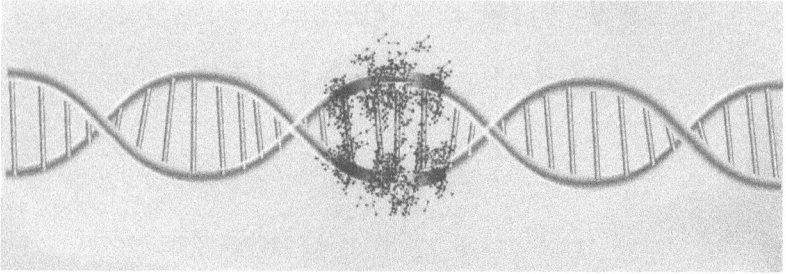

Figure 1: Human DNA molecules

OXYGEN AND FOOD:

When chemicals in food are exposed to Oxygen, their chemical composition changes, and they biodegrade at a faster rate than normal. However, animal and plant tissues contain antioxidant molecules that can inhibit this process and delay the oxidation rate in our foods [7]. However, antioxidant molecules have a limited capacity, and prolonged exposure to free radicals reduces food's nutritional value and induce an early onset of discoloration and biodegradation. The oxidation of food proteins reduces their nutritional value and may introduce contamination and infections. Protein oxidation can significantly induce degenerative reactions to muscle foods, which generally contain 17 to 25 percent of protein in their raw or unprepared form [8]. Protein oxidation is usually related to other oxidation reactions in foods, such as lipid oxidation and enzymatic reactions where oxygen serves as a catalyst. However, not much attention has been paid to protein oxidation since the oxidation pathways are more complex, the form of the oxidative products are more significant, and the effects and discernible consequences are usually less noticeable by consumers.

Oxidative mutation in the protein component of muscle foods occurs when free radicals are created, which can induce protein crosslinking, amino acid side-chain modification, and protein fragmentation [8]. It is well established that certain amino acids and proteins are more susceptible to forming free radicals than others. For example, myoglobin, an essential protein in the skeletal muscle, is highly vulnerable to protein oxidation, which induces alterations in colour and reduced quality of meat. Protein oxidation is a complex process that needs in-depth scientific research at the intermediary level.

Several intrinsic and extrinsic factors increase the susceptibility of muscle foods to protein oxidation [9]. Intrinsic factors include the animal species, the origin of the animal, genetics and environmental factors during production, the muscle type, and the product's composition. The extrinsic factors include the processing conditions, the packaging conditions, and even the preparation proficiency or techniques [8, 9].Various laboratory techniques to quantify the degree of protein oxidation in meat products include indirect analytical methods. These methods focus on measuring and evaluating the formation and level of reactivity of carbonyls, the formation, and level of reactivity of carbonyl derivatives, the modification of amino acid side chains, the formation of protein crosslinks, and the assemblage or polymerisation of proteins [1].

There are limitations to each of these techniques, as they are time-dependent, necessitate a detailed protocol, and sometimes demand the standardization of a working protocol. The most routinely used technique to measure protein oxidation is the analysis of carbonyl derivatives, primarily the derivatisation of protein carbonyls with 2,4-dinitrophenylhydrazine (DNPH) to produce a DNPH complex [10]. This complex can be detected with high-performance liquid chromatography (HPLC) and mass spectrometry. The advantages of this and similar techniques are an abundance of protein carbonyls in a given tissue for easy detection. In contrast, other methods, such as quantifying sulfhydryl groups, are only effective for proteins with a significant number of amino acids with sulfur groups, cysteine, or methionine. Additionally, several novel laboratory techniques are being developed to detect protein oxidation in muscle foods.

THE OUTCOMES OF OXIDATION

As outlined in earlier sections, a significant level of complexity in reactions and interactions exists during oxidation, and a broad range of factors influence this process. Thus, it is almost impossible to tell the extent of oxidation in food and biological products. However, several analytical methods targeting various markers of oxidation have been developed. The oxidative process results in several outcomes, including the loss of protein elements, such as tryptophan and sulfhydryl groups, and the formation of oxidation products, such as protein carbonyls and crosslinks, which collectively cause cell death (figure 2).

Oxidation occurs in muscle foods, such as fresh and processed fish and meat products [9]. Unlike lipid oxidation which is generally well-described in the science-based community, protein oxidation is less recognised due to its invisible effect on flavour and colour of food [3]. Naturally, the proteins in foods can be oxidised by the direct reactions with reactive Oxygen and nitrogen species or an indirect induction from oxidative by-products of sugars and lipids [11]. Although research has provided a general overview of oxidation reactions in meat products, there is still a shortage of systematic and in-depth literature about the outcomes and mechanism of protein oxidation. Therefore, a better understanding of the outcome of oxidation and the protein reaction process, as well as the classification of protein oxidation such as photo-oxidation, metal-catalyzed protein oxidation, and enzyme-catalyzed protein oxidation, is critical in understanding the outcome of oxidation on our healthspan and lifespan

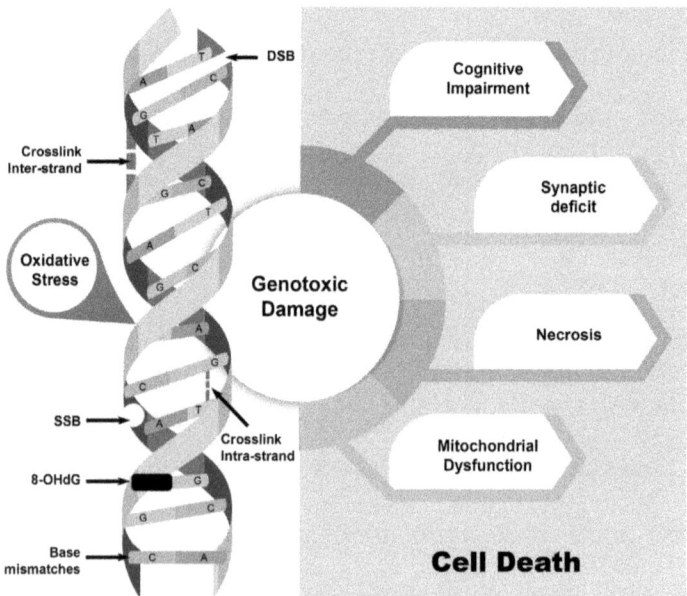

Figure 2: Cell death due to an excess of free radicals, called oxidative stress.

CHAPTER TWO

Roles of Free Radicals in Our Body Systems

Free radicals are the products of cellular metabolism and can be defined as an atom or molecule with one or more unpaired electrons in a valence shell or an outer orbit and can exist independently. The odd number of electrons in a free radical makes it unstable, short-lived, and highly reactive with surrounding molecules of DNA, proteins, and lipids. As a result of their high reactivity, free radicals can extract electrons from surrounding molecules to achieve stability. Thus, the attacked molecule loses its electron and subsequently becomes a free radical, creating a chain reaction that irreversibly damages the living cell. Our cells have an antioxidant defense system to contain free radicals [12]. However, in excess production, free radicals can severely damage cells, tissues, and organs [13].

Reactive Oxygen Species (ROS) and Reactive Nitrogen Species (RNS) are the prominent free radicals in our cells. The ROS/RNS play a double-fold role as both beneficial and toxic elements to the living system. At moderate or low levels, ROS/RNS have protective effects and regulate several physiological functions of the body, such as immune function-defense against pathogenic microorganisms in many cellular signaling pathways, redox regulation, and mitogenic response [14]. However, at higher concentrations, ROS and RNS generate oxidative and nitrosative stress, respectively, which damage several biomolecules in the cells, including DNA, lipids, and proteins [5]. Oxidative and nitrosative stress occurs when there is an excess production of reactive Oxygen and nitrogen species beyond the capacity of cellular antioxidant systems to handle them. Most importantly, the excess reactive oxygen and nitrogen species can damage the integrity of several biomolecules, including lipids, proteins, and DNA, contributing to increased oxidative stress (figure 3).

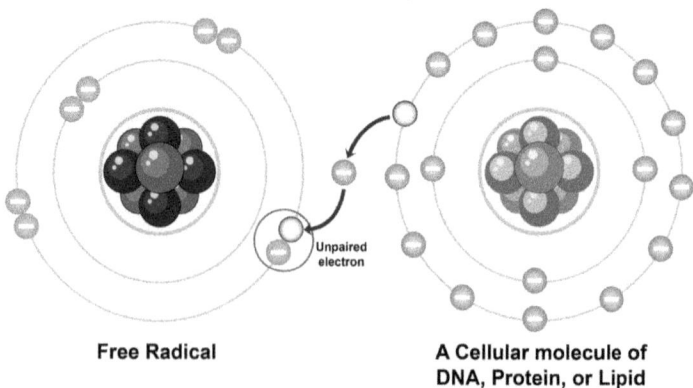

Free Radical   **A Cellular molecule of DNA, Protein, or Lipid**

Figure 3: The mechanism of action of free radicals.

Several lines of evidence indicate the critical roles of elevated oxidative stress in human diseases, such as rheumatoid arthritis, diabetes mellitus, neurodegenerative diseases, cataracts, cardiovascular diseases, respiratory diseases and accelerating your ageing process [12, 15-17].

REACTIVE OXYGEN SPECIES (ROS) AND REACTIVE NITROGEN SPECIES (RNS):

Free radicals are the species with at least one unpaired electron in the shells around the atomic nucleus and can exist independently [18]. The oxygen molecule is a radical, and due to the presence of two unpaired electrons, it is called "biradical." Examples of radicals species include Oxygen radical ($O\cdot\cdot2$), Hydroxyl ($OH\cdot$), Alkoxyradical ($RO\cdot$), Superoxide ($O\cdot-2$), Peroxyl radical ($ROO\cdot$), Nitric oxide or nitrogen monoxide ($NO\cdot$), and nitrogen dioxide ($NO\cdot2$).

The high reactivity of these radicals stems from the presence of one unpaired electron, which donates or obtains another electron to attain stability. The non-radical species include hydrogen peroxide ($H2O2$), ozone ($O3$), hypochlorous acid ($HOCl$), singlet oxygen

(1O2), hypobromous acid (HOBr), nitrous acid (HNO2), dinitrogen trioxide (N2O3), nitrosyl cation (NO+), nitroxyl anion (NO−), organic peroxides (ROOH), dinitrogen tetraoxide (N2O4), nitronium (nitryl) cation (NO2+), aldehydes (HCOR) and peroxynitrite (ONOOH). Although they are not free radicals, the non-radical species can easily cause free radical reactions in living organisms. The half-life of some radicals depends on the environmental factor; for instance, the half-life of nitric oxide (NO•) in an air-saturated solution may be a few minutes.

HISTORY OF RESEARCH ON FREE RADICALS:

In recent years, there has been a rapidly growing interest in evaluating the role of free radicals in biology due to their significant role in various physiological conditions and their involvement in several diseases. In 1900, Moses Gomberg, a Professor of Chemistry at the University of Michigan, hypothesised the existence of an organic free radical, triphenyl methyl radical (Ph3C•), in a biological or living system. Subsequently, in 1954, Gershman propounded the "free radical theory of oxygen toxicity," where he proposed that an excess of free radicals and oxygen toxicity contribute to the ageing process in humans [19]. In the same year, the study of electron paramagnetic resonance (EPR) by Commoner et al. 1954 verified the existence of free radicals in biological materials [20]. Shortly after that, in 1956, Denham Harman proposed the "free radical theory of ageing," which states that free radicals play a pivotal role in the ageing process [19]. The second era of free radical studies began in 1969 with McCord and Fridovich, who found the superoxide dismutase, the first enzymatic defense system against superoxide anion [21].

In 1971, Loschen illustrated that the Reactive oxygen species are produced in cellular metabolic respiration, which was later validated and expanded by Nohl and Hegner in 1978 [22]. In 1977, Mittal and Murad observed that the hydroxyl radical OH˙ causes the formation of the second messenger cyclic GMP by activating the enzyme guanylate cyclase [23]. In 1989, Halliwell and Gutteridge stated that reactive oxygen species (ROS) include free radical and non-radical derivatives of Oxygen [24]. From that period, massive data has been generated on the role of free radicals in various pathophysiological conditions.

THE ACTION OF FREE RADICALS AND THEIR EFFECT ON CELL HEALTH:

Free radicals are unstable atoms that can induce diseases and accelerate the ageing process by damaging cellular molecules. Free radicals are associated with ageing and many diseases, though little is uncovered about their role in human health [25]. In general, an excess of free radicals damage cellular DNA, proteins, and lipids, which collectively causes cellular damage and dysfunction (figure 4).

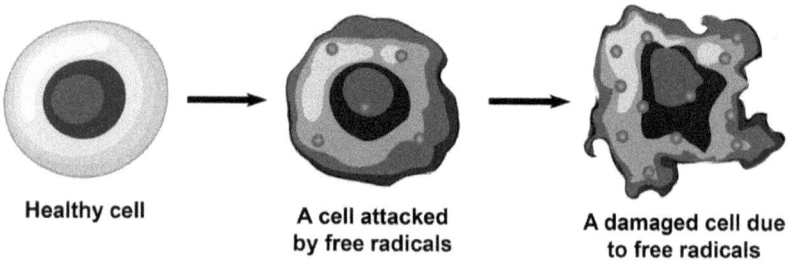

Healthy cell   **A cell attacked by free radicals**   **A damaged cell due to free radicals**

Figure 4: The effects of free radicals on human body cells.

Since these cells exist as components of our body tissues and organs, the cumulative result is the diseases of specific organs. Some of the diseases associated with free radicals include:

- Inflammation of the joints (arthritis)
- Certain cancers are caused by damage to DNA of cells
- Impairment of the eye lens, which contributes to loss of vision

- Increased risk of coronary heart disease by causing low-density lipoprotein (LDL) cholesterol to stick to artery walls
- Brain nerve cells damage contributes to conditions such as Parkinson's or Alzheimer's disease
- Acceleration of the ageing process

Free radicals are also responsible for age-related changes in our external appearance, including wrinkles and grey hair. Understanding the effect of free radicals requires a basic knowledge of chemistry since atoms are bordered by electrons that orbit the atom in layers called shells, and a set number of electrons must fill each shell [1]. When a shell is complete, the electrons start filling the next shell. If an atom has an outer shell that is not full, it may bond with another atom and utilize the electrons to complete its outer shell. These types of atoms are termed free radicals.

Though atoms with an entire outer shell are stable, free radicals are unstable, and in trying to complete the number of electrons in their outer shell, they quickly react with other substances. When oxygen molecules split into single atoms with unpaired electrons, they become unstable free radicals that search for other atoms or molecules to bond with. We call it oxidative stress if there is a higher than normal level of free radicals in the cell [26]. Oxidative stress can damage your body cells, tissues, and organs and exacerbate the natural ageing process, such as the early appearance of grey hairs and wrinkles.

MECHANISM OF CELLULAR DAMAGE BY FREE RADICALS

Free radicals are unstable atoms, and to be stable, they extract electrons from other atoms, which contributes to diseases or early ageing [16, 27]. According to the free radical theory of ageing, which was first proposed in 1956, free radicals biodegrade cells over time [19]. As the body ages, its antioxidant systems and the ability to offset the effects of free radicals decline, which contributes to higher levels of free radicals, increased oxidative stress, and more damage to cells, which collectively accelerate the natural degenerative ageing processes [11].

Several studies support the free radical theory of ageing. For example, the research on laboratory rats shows a significant increase in free radicals as they age, which mirrors the age-related deterioration in the systemic health of the rats [28]. Over time, researchers have modified the free radical theory of ageing to focus on the mitochondria, which are cellular powerhouses and produce energy by using oxygen [16]. Research on rats proposed that the mitochondria's free radicals damage the substances the cell needs to function correctly. This damage causes changes that produce more free radicals, thus further damaging the cell. This theory best explains the symptoms of ageing since ageing accelerates over time with the activities of free radicals. The gradual yet increasingly rapid accumulation of free radicals offers an insight into why even healthy bodies age and decline over time.

EFFECTS OF OXIDATIVE STRESS ON THE BODY:

Oxidation is a typical chemical reaction in our cells. However, oxidative stress, characterized by higher levels of free radicals, can damage our bodies. A few free radicals can help fight off pathogens known for causing infections. However, when there is a higher production of free radicals beyond the capacity of antioxidant systems to stabilise them, the free radicals can start causing damage to fatty tissue, DNA, and the proteins in your body [11]. Proteins, lipids, and DNA comprise a large part of your body. Thus, damage can cause many diseases over time, such as:

- Heart disease

- Inflammatory conditions

- Diabetes

- Cancer

- Atherosclerosis, or the hardening of the blood vessels

- Neurodegenerative diseases, such as Parkinson's and Alzheimer's diseases

- High blood pressure, also called hypertension

- Oxidative stress, which also contributes to ageing

NEUTRALIZATION OF FREE RADICALS

Free radicals have lost electrons and become unstable. Hence, they can be stabilised by receiving electrons. Though free radicals and antioxidants are part of the body's natural and healthy functioning, oxidative stress occurs when there is an imbalance between the levels of free radicals and antioxidants. Oxidative stress can cause damage to many tissues, contributing to several diseases over time. Though the production of free radicals cannot be prevented, lifestyle choices, such as a healthy diet, exercise, and a healthy lifestyle, can minimize the levels of free radicals in the body, preventing diseases and early ageing [29].

We all naturally produce some free radicals in our bodies through exercise or inflammation. A small number of free radicals are essential to the body's system for keeping itself healthy. There are many ways you can be exposed to free radicals in the environment, such as:

- Pollution
- Cigarette smoke
- Ozone
- Certain pesticides and cleaners
- A diet that is high in sugar, fat, and alcohol may also contribute to free radical production.
- Radiation

STABILISING AND NEUTRALISING OXIDATIVE STRESS:

It is impossible to completely stop the production of free radicals and oxidative stress. However, there are ways to minimise the effects of oxidative stress on your body systems. For example, antioxidant molecules can effectively neutralize free radicals in our cells. Thus, an intake of food rich in antioxidants can reduce the formation of free radicals and make us healthy [29]. You can neutralise oxidative stress by obtaining adequate antioxidants in your diet. Antioxidants are present in certain foods and may reverse some of the damage caused by free radicals by neutralising them. Common antioxidants include vitamins A, C, and E, and the minerals copper, zinc, and Selenium in your diet. Similarly, dietary food compounds, such as the phytochemicals in plants, have more potent antioxidant properties than vitamins or minerals [30, 31]. Though they are called non-nutrient antioxidants, they include phytochemicals, such as lycopene in tomatoes and anthocyanins present in cranberries.

Eating five daily servings of various fruits and vegetables is an incredible way to boost your body's ability to produce antioxidants. Examples of fruits and vegetables rich in antioxidants include:

- Dark leafy greens
- Olives
- Broccoli
- Citrus fruits
- Prunes
- Carrots
- Berries
- Cherries
- Tomatoes

Other examples of dietary antioxidant sources include:

- Vitamin C

- Vitamin E

- Nuts

- Garlic

- Turmeric

- Melatonin

- Green tea

- Fish

- Cinnamon

- Onion

Other healthy lifestyle choices can also stabilise or neutralise oxidative stress. Below are some beneficial lifestyle changes to prevent oxidative stress:

- Avoid smoking and exposure to secondhand smoke [32].

- **A regular and moderate workout routine:** It has been linked with increased natural antioxidant levels and reduction of damage induced by oxidative stress. Regular exercise is associated with a longer lifespan, lesser impacts of ageing, and reduced risk of cancer and disease [33].

- **Be cautious with chemicals:** Be cautious of cleaning agents and other chemicals. Avoid unnecessary radiation exposure, and be conscious of other chemical exposure sources, including pesticides used on food or gardening.

- Wear sunscreen in daylight and prevent ultraviolet light from damaging your skin.

- Reduce your alcohol intake.

- **Get adequate sleep:** An optimal amount of sleep is essential for vitality and maintaining balance in your body systems. Your brain function, hormone production, muscle recovery, skin nourishment, antioxidant and free radical balance, and many other things are negatively affected by lack of sleep.

- **Avoid overfeeding:** Several food studies have discovered that overeating keeps your body in a state of oxidative stress more often than eating in small or moderate portions at appropriately timed and spaced intervals.

Therefore, if **oxidation** produces potentially harmful agents, called **free radicals, neutralising** the bad outcomes requires an **antioxidant**.

CHAPTER THREE

Introduction to Antioxidants [Vit ADECKSe], Se=selenium:

O xidation creates unstable chemicals called free radicals, which damage various cellular structures and are linked to developing several diseases, including heart disease, liver disorders, and neurodegenerative diseases [12, 15, 17]. Antioxidants are compounds in foods that fight and neutralise these free radicals (figure 5). Antioxidants such as thiols or ascorbic acid (vitamin C) may help neutralise the free radicals in the cells [29].

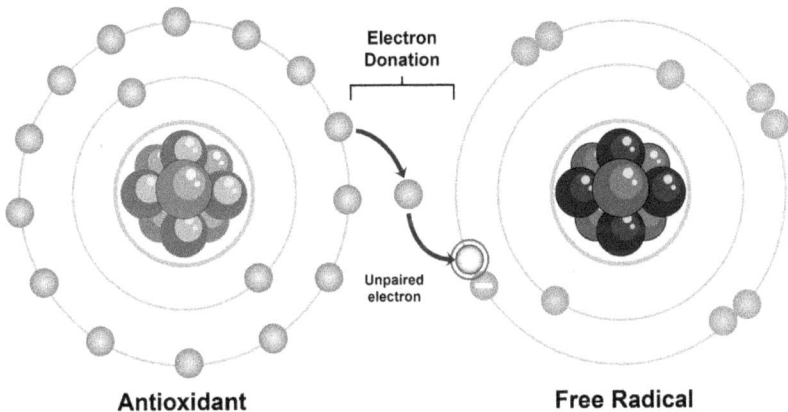

Figure 5: Mechanism of action through which antioxidants neutralize free radicals.

A diet high in antioxidants reduces the risk of many diseases, including heart disease and certain cancers.

Here are some antioxidants, food sources, and their chemical properties (figure 6):

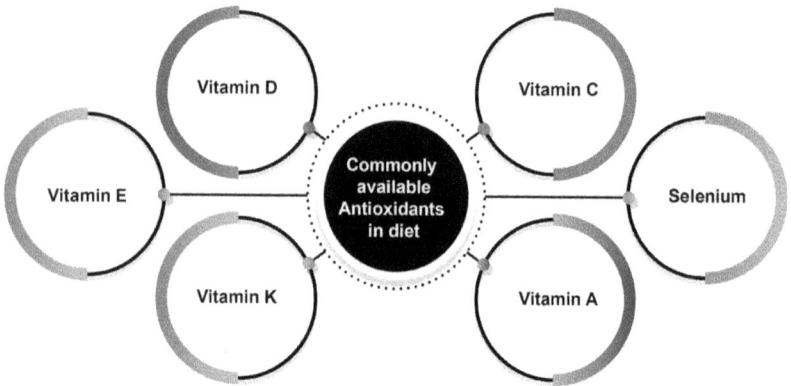

Figure 6: Antioxidants in diet

I. **Vitamin A:** It is one of the essential micronutrients and is integral for many vital functions such as epithelial integrity, cell growth, and immune system response. Vitamin A also has anti-infectious properties due to its critical role in immune function by regulating the differentiation of T-helper cells (TH1-TH2), Th2 production of interleukin-4 and interleukin-5, controlling the humoral antibody response, and inhibition of bacteria growth [34]. Vitamin A also operates as an antioxidant agent, impeding oxidative stress and cell damage. The antioxidant action of vitamin A and carotenoids is bestowed by the hydrophobic chain of polyene units that can suppress singlet oxygen, neutralise thiyl radicals and combine with and stabilise peroxyl radicals. Generally, the longer the polyene chain, the higher the Peroxyl radical stabilising ability. Vitamin A is found in several food sources, such as green and yellow vegetables, dairy products (beef liver, lamb liver, etc.), salmon, cod liver oil, butter, goat cheese, trout, fruits, and organ meats which are some of the richest sources [35]. In the body, it can be found as retinol, retinal and retinoic acid. Since a higher amount of vitamin A is toxic to cells, it is found in a form bound to proteins in the extracellular fluids and inside cells. Vitamin A is stored typically as long-chain fatty esters and as pro-vitamin carotenoids in the kidney, liver, and adipose tissue. Due to their structures, vitamin A and carotenoids can autoxidise when O2 tension rises. Therefore, they are the most beneficial antioxidants at low oxygen tensions, which are found at an average physiological level in the tissues. Epidemiological evidence suggests that vitamin A and carotenoids are vital dietary factors for reducing the occurrence of heart and skin diseases [36].

II. **Vitamin D:** It is a natural and membrane antioxidant. Therefore, vitamin D3 (cholecalciferol) and its active metabolite 1,25-dihydroxycholecalciferol, vitamin D2 (ergocalciferol), and 7-dehydrocholesterol (pro-Vitamin D3) all impede iron-dependent liposomal lipid peroxidation [26]. The structural rationale for the antioxidant ability of these Vitamin D compounds is considered based on their molecular relationship to cholesterol and ergosterol. The antioxidant ability of Vitamin D is correlated with the anti-cancer drug tamoxifen and its 4-hydroxy metabolite. Vitamin D is a natural antioxidant that has evidence of anti-cancer action, improving antioxidant enzyme levels in COPD and asthma, but not in ACO patients (has asthma and COPD). Vitamin D (Vit D) does not only contribute to sustaining normal calcium metabolism, but it is also crucial for a substantial extent of non-classic actions. The antioxidant effects of Vit D are linked to the non-calcemic roles of this compound. Vitamin D deficiency is associated with several chronic diseases, such as diabetes and cardiovascular and chronic kidney disease (CKD), and skin disorders [36]. It can be found in oily fish, red meat, liver, egg yolks, etc [37].

III. **Vitamin E:** It is a potent chain-breaking antioxidant that restrains the production of reactive oxygen species molecules when fat undergoes oxidation and multiplication of free radical reactions [38]. It is primarily located in the cell and organelle membranes, where it can maintain its optimal protective effect, even when its concentration ratio is only one molecule for every 2,000 phospholipid molecules. It is the first defense against lipid peroxidation, defending the cell membranes from free radical attack. Vitamin E optimizes the packaging of membrane lipids in the sarcolemma of cells. Therefore, permitting tighter packing of the membrane and, in turn, more stellar stability to the cell. In 2011, Howard et al. observed that vitamin E is essential for maintaining proper skeletal muscle homeostasis and that the supplementation of cultured myocytes with alpha-tocopherol encourages plasma membrane repair. This occurs because the membrane phospholipids are high targets of oxidants, and vitamin E efficiently inhibits lipid peroxidation. It can be found in sunflower seeds, red bell pepper, pumpkin, almonds, wheat germ oil, peanuts, peanut butter, etc.

IV. **Vitamin C:** As an antioxidant, it fights against oxidative stress-induced cellular damage by neutralising reactive oxygen species, vitamin E-dependent counteraction of lipid hydroperoxyl radicals, and defending proteins from alkylation by electrophilic lipid peroxidation products [36]. Vitamin C (ascorbic acid) is an essential cofactor for α-ketoglutarate-dependent dioxygenases. Examples are prolyl hydroxylases, which contribute to the biosynthesis of collagen and in the downregulation of hypoxia-inducible factor (HIF)-1, a transcription factor that regulates several genes responsible for energy metabolism, tumour growth, and neutrophil function and apoptosis [39]. Vitamin C-dependent inhibition of the HIF pathway may offer an alternative for regulating tumour progression, infections, and inflammation. Vitamin E (α-tocopherol) functions as a crucial lipid-soluble antioxidant, inhibiting hydroperoxyl radicals in the lipid environment. Any symptoms of vitamin E deficiency in humans hint that its antioxidant effects significantly protect nervous tissues and erythrocyte membranes [40]. Moreover, Vitamin C also has a role in endothelial nitric oxide synthase (eNOS) activity by recycling the eNOS cofactor, tetrahydrobiopterin, which is crucial to arterial elasticity and blood pressure regulation. It is naturally found in potatoes, walnuts, strawberries, brussel sprouts, pepper, broccoli, oranges, etc.

V. **Vitamin K:** It has antioxidant properties and protects cellular membranes from damage due to the availability of excess free radicals [41]. This process is called peroxidation. Blood thinning medication like warfarin can reduce the anti-oxidative properties of Vitamin K. Vitamins K-1 and K-2 have distinct chemical structures, and both have a phytyl side chain, but K-2 also possesses isoprenoid side chains. K-2 has many subtypes, called menaquinones (MKs), numbered MK-4 to MK-13, depending on the length of their side chains. K-1 is the typical form of the vitamin, and it is typically found in leafy green vegetables. However, the body finds it difficult to absorb vitamin K-1 from plants. The body necessitates both types of vitamin K to create prothrombin, a protein that plays essential roles in bone metabolism, blood clotting, and heart health [41]. Vitamin K also assists in energy production in the mitochondria of cells. It is naturally found in blueberries, soybean, lettuces, canola oil, broccoli, spinach, etc [42].

VI. **Selenium:** Antioxidants like Selenium reduce oxidative stress by regulating free radicals. They function by neutralising excess free radicals and protecting the cells from damage induced by oxidative stress [43]. Selenium (Se) is an essential trace element, and its low quantity in humans has been correlated to a higher risk of various diseases, such as heart disease and cancer [44]. Recently, Selenium research has received tremendous interest due to its integral role in antioxidant selenoproteins for defense against oxidative stress induced by excess reactive oxygen species (ROS) and reactive nitrogen species (NOS). The synthesis of selenoproteins requires a distinct internalisation of amino acid selenocysteine (Sec) into proteins regulated by the UGA codon, which is also a termination codon. This interest in Selenium research has contributed to the discovery of at least 30 selenoproteins. However, the biochemical, and functional roles of some selenoproteins are still unclear. Apart from the form of selenoproteins, Se can be found in several other chemical forms in biological materials either as organic Se compounds like selenomethionine and dimethylselenide, and inorganic compounds like selenites and selenates. In foods, Se is predominantly found as selenomethionine, an essential source of dietary Se in humans, and also as a chemical form commonly adopted for Se supplements in clinical trials. The possibility for deficiency diseases linked with low Selenium status has contributed to the formation of the recommended daily requirements for Selenium in many countries. However, excess Selenium intake through supplementation and its potential abuse as health therapy could also become a risk factor for developing different diseases. As an essential trace element, the vitality of Selenium in humans is well documented, and its deficiency has caused adverse health effects in humans, such as Keshan disease. Foods are the typical and natural source of Selenium, and its levels generally depend on soil Selenium levels. Since its discovery as an essential component of antioxidant enzymes, such as thioredoxin reductase (TrxR), glutathione peroxidase (GPx), and iodothyronine deiodinases (IDD), a rapid interest has developed in the study of other Selenium-containing proteins, such as selenoproteins, or enzymes such as selenoenzymes. It can be found in Brazil nuts, eggs, red meat, poultry, bread, seafood, organ meats, etc.

DIETARY RECOMMENDATIONS FOR ANTIOXIDANTS:

There are conflicting reports on whether antioxidant supplements provide the same health benefits as food antioxidants. Evidence shows that antioxidant supplements don't work like the naturally occurring antioxidants in fruits and vegetables. To have a healthy and well-balanced diet, it is recommended that you consume a variety of foods from the main five food groups daily:

- Whole grain foods and cereals
- Vegetables
- Legumes
- Fruit
- Beans
- Lean meat
- Poultry or alternatives such as fish, tofu, legumes, eggs, nuts, and seeds
- Dairy and dairy alternatives primarily reduce fat, though reduced fat milk is not recommended for children below two years.

Aim to eat at least a single daily serving of fruit and vegetables to meet your nutritional requirements. Although serving sizes vary depending on weight, sex, age, and stage of life, this is approximately a medium-sized piece of fruit or a half-cup of cooked vegetables. The Australian Dietary Guidelines provide further information on recommended servings and portions for specific ages, gender, and life stage. It is also proposed that antioxidants and other protective ingredients from vegetables, legumes, and fruit must be regularly consumed from early life to be effective [29, 36]. Consult your healthcare provider or dietitian for assistance and advice.

CHEMICAL UNIQUENESS OF ANTIOXIDANTS

Antioxidants are compounds that neutralise oxidation—a chemical reaction that can generate free radicals that can damage your body cells. Antioxidants such as thiols or ascorbic acid (vitamin C) may help to neutralise these reactions. A diet high in antioxidants reduces the risk of developing several diseases, including heart disease and certain cancers [45]. The protective effect and chemical distinction of antioxidants are a subject of ongoing global research. For instance, men who consume plenty of the antioxidant lycopene found in red fruits and vegetables like watermelon, tomatoes, apricots, and pink grapefruit may exhibit reduced susceptibility to developing prostate cancer [46]. Lycopene consumption reduces the risk of developing type 2 diabetes mellitus. Lutein found in corn and spinach has been linked to a lower risk of eye lens degeneration and vision loss in the elderly [47]. Research also hints that dietary lutein may enhance memory and neutralise cognitive decline [47]. Several research studies have found that flavonoid-rich foods inhibit many diseases, including cancer and metabolic-related diseases. Apples, grapes, berries, tea, olive oil, citrus fruits, onions, and red wine are the most commonly used sources of flavonoids.

CHEMICAL STRUCTURE OF AN ANTIOXIDANT

An antioxidant is a substance that prevents substrate oxidation by neutralizing free radicals in the cell. Antioxidant compounds use several chemical mechanisms, such as single electron transfer (SET), hydrogen atom transfer (HAT), and the ability to chelate transition metals. The essence of antioxidant mechanisms is to comprehend the biological implication of antioxidants, their unique structure, their production by organic synthesis or biotechnological techniques, or the standardisation for determining antioxidant activity.

Generally, antioxidant molecules react either by diverse mechanisms or by a predominant mechanism. The chemical structure of the antioxidant substance gives an insight into the antioxidant reaction mechanism. This section reviews the in-vitro antioxidant reaction mechanisms and uniqueness of organic compounds such as polyphenols, carotenoids, and vitamins C against free radicals (FR) and pro-oxidant compounds under various health conditions and diseases. Additionally, the antioxidant activities of these compounds are discussed according to the mechanism involved in the reaction with free radicals [7]. The prominent uniqueness of antioxidants is the ability to prevent or detect a chain of oxidative propagation by stabilising the generated radical, thereby reducing oxidative damage in the human body.

Gordon classified antioxidants into two main types: the primary antioxidants, which neutralises the chain reaction. The secondary antioxidant mechanisms may include the regeneration of primary antioxidants, the deactivation of metals, inhibition of lipid hydroperoxides by inhibiting the production of unwanted volatiles, and the liquidation of singlet oxygen [48]. Hence, antioxidants can be described as those substances that, in low quantities, act by preventing or decelerating the oxidation of easily oxidisable materials, such as fats.

ROLE OF ANTIOXIDANTS:

Biological systems in oxygenated environments have in-built defense mechanisms, such as physiological and biochemical. At the physiological level is a micro-vascular system that sustains the levels of O2 in the tissues. At the biochemical level, the antioxidant defense can be enzymatic or non-enzymatic and serve as a system for repairing molecules.

I. **Primary enzymatic system:** Aerobic organisms have engendered antioxidant enzymes, such as glutathione peroxidase (GPx), superoxide dismutase (SOD), catalase (CAT), and DT-diaphorase. Superoxide dismutase is responsible for the dis-mutation reaction of O2 to H2O2, which in subsequent reactions is catalysed by catalase or GPx and converted into harmless H2O and O2. SOD is the most essential and potent detoxification enzyme in the cell [49]. SOD is a metalloenzyme and needs a metal as a cofactor for its activity. Based on the type of metal ion required as a cofactor by superoxide dismutase, there are many forms of the enzyme [49]. Catalase uses iron or manganese as a cofactor. It catalyses the reduction of hydrogen peroxide (H2O2) to water and molecular Oxygen, thereby completing the detoxification process initiated by superoxide dismutase [50]. Catalase is highly efficient in biodegrading millions of H2O2 molecules in a second.

II. CAT is mainly present in peroxisomes, and its primary function is to decimate the H2O2 generated during the oxidation of fatty acids [50]. Glutathione peroxidase is an essential intracellular enzyme that breaks down H2O2 in water and lipid peroxides in their corresponding alcohols, primarily in mitochondria [51]. The activity of glutathione peroxidase depends on Selenium. There are about eight isoforms of glutathione peroxidase in humans, namely GPx1–GPx8. Among glutathione peroxidases, GPx1 is the most luxuriant selenoperoxidase found in nearly all cells [51]. The enzyme is essential in neutralising lipid peroxidation and protects cells from oxidative stress. Low GPx activity causes oxidative damage to the cell membrane's functional proteins and fatty acids. Glutathione peroxidase, especially GPx1, has been culpably involved in developing and preventing many diseases, including cancer and cardiovascular diseases. DT-diaphorase catalyses the decrease of quinone to quinol and helps reduce drugs of quinone structure. However, DNA determines the production of these enzymes in cells.

III. **Non-enzymatic system:** This contains antioxidants that trap free radicals and prevent radical initiation. They do so by donating electrons and are consequently transformed into free radicals, albeit with less reactivity than the initial free radical. Other antioxidants easily neutralise free radicals from antioxidants in this group. The cells use a variety of antioxidant compounds or free radical scavengers, such as vitamin C, vitamin E, ceruloplasmin, carotenes, ferritin, Selenium, reduced glutathione (GSH), manganese, ubiquinone, zinc, flavonoids, coenzyme Q, bilirubin, taurine, melatonin, and cysteine. The flavonoids from certain foods directly interact with reactive species to create stable complexes or complexes with less reactivity. In contrast, in other foods, the flavonoids function as co-substrate in the catalytic action of some enzymes.

IV. **Repair system:** Enzymes that repair or inhibit the biomolecules damaged by reactive oxidative species, such as proteins, lipids, and DNA, comprise the repair systems. Typical examples are systems of **DNA repair enzymes** like glycosylases, polymerases, and nucleases, and **proteolytic enzymes** like proteases, proteinases, and peptidases in the cytosol and the mitochondria of mammalian cells. These enzymes are glutathione peroxidases, glutathione reductase (GR), and methionine sulfoxide reductase (MSR) [51]. These enzymes act as intercessors in the repair process of oxidative damage caused by the production of excess reactive oxidative species. Any environmental factor that inhibits or mutates a regular biological activity favours the occurrence or reinforcement of oxidative stress.

THE IMPORTANCE OF THE EXCESS ELECTRONS

Antioxidants are substances that can protect your cells against free radicals, which contribute to heart disease, cancer, and other diseases [45]. Free radicals are highly reactive molecules created due to a breakdown of food or exposure to radiation, pollution, or tobacco smoke. Excess electrons neutralise free radicals or stabilise them by donating electrons, which converts the antioxidants into free radicals. Though, they will be less reactive than the initial free radicals.

PRINCIPLE OF THE ANTIOXIDANT WAY TO LIVING LONGER:

Free radical theories of ageing and disease provide insight into why some people age more slowly than others. Although free radicals are naturally produced in the body, several lifestyle and environmental factors can increase their production [19]. These lifestyle factors have been associated with diseases such as cancer and cardiovascular disease. Hence, oxidative stress might be the reason exposure to substances causes disease. Free radicals are oxygen-containing molecules with an uneven or odd number of electrons, allowing them to react with other molecules efficiently. Free radicals can cause large-chain chemical reactions because they react readily with other molecules. These reactions can be beneficial or harmful.

Research examining the relationship between oxidation and ageing is growing. According to various ageing models, research has found that dietary calorie restriction and some antioxidants can extend lifespan. Oxygen is crucial to aerobic organisms since it is a final electron acceptor in mitochondria. However, Oxygen is harmful due to its ability to continuously generate reactive oxygen species (ROS), which can induce or exacerbate the process of ageing [19]. To remove these ROS in cells, aerobic organisms have an antioxidant defense system that comprises a series of enzymes, such as superoxide dismutase (SOD), catalase (CAT), glutathione peroxidase (GPx), and glutathione reductase (GR) [5]. Additionally, dietary antioxidants such as vitamin A, vitamin C, α-tocopherol, ascorbic acid, and plant flavonoids can neutralise ROS in cells and improve our healthspan [52]. Additionally, animal studies indicate that prolonged supplementation of antioxidants can increase lifespan in laboratory rodents. For example, vitamin E, some phytochemicals, royal jelly, and some enzymes delivered through genes can significantly extend the lifespan of mice and rats [53-57]. In addition, a considerable improvement in healthspan is also reported as evident by improved kidney, liver, and cognitive functions [53, 56]. However, these results should be interpreted cautiously since the effects of antioxidants on lifespan are not always consistent [57].

Antioxidants help stabilise cells and protect them from oxidative stress, which can cause cancer, heart disease, and eye diseases like age-related macular degeneration [14]. Scientists have proposed that antioxidants help support longevity based on the free radical theory of ageing [19]. However, more recent research indicates that the actual cause of ageing is much more complex.

Free radicals destroy DNA, but antioxidants inhibit them from destroying the DNA. Hence, the DNA's integrity is maintained, and its lifespan is extended. According to Marisa Moore, RDN, based in Atlanta, antioxidants help inhibit or slow damage to our cells. Vitamin C may help prevent or delay certain cancers and support healthy ageing.

PHYTOCHEMICALS

Phytochemical is a broad term for chemicals and a wide variety of compounds that are naturally found in plants [58]. The phytochemicals are classified into six primary categories depending on their chemical structures and characteristics. These categories include carbohydrates, terpenoids, lipids, phenolics, alkaloids, and other nitrogen-containing compounds

Phytochemicals capable of providing health benefits are carotenoids, polyphenols, flavonoids, isoflavonoids, anthocyanidins, phytoestrogens, terpenoids, limonoids, glucosinolates, phytosterols, and fibres. Several bioactive phytochemicals are found in commonly consumed plant foods, such as fruits, spices, vegetables, and beverages [58]. Their presence in the diet and low toxicity hint that phytochemicals can affect human health and disease risk at the population level.

When considering bioavailability, dietary phytochemicals can be categorised into two distinct classes:

- Water-soluble phytochemicals, such as phenolics and poly-phenols.

- Lipid-soluble phytochemicals, such as carotenoids, curcum-inoids, and tocochromanols.

MOST POPULAR DRINKS AND FOODS THAT ARE TOUTED AS RICH IN ANTIOXIDANTS AND WHY:

Many natural foods contain at least some quantities of antioxidants, though Taylor Wolfram, RDN, states that fruits and vegetables are the best sources of antioxidants (figure 7).

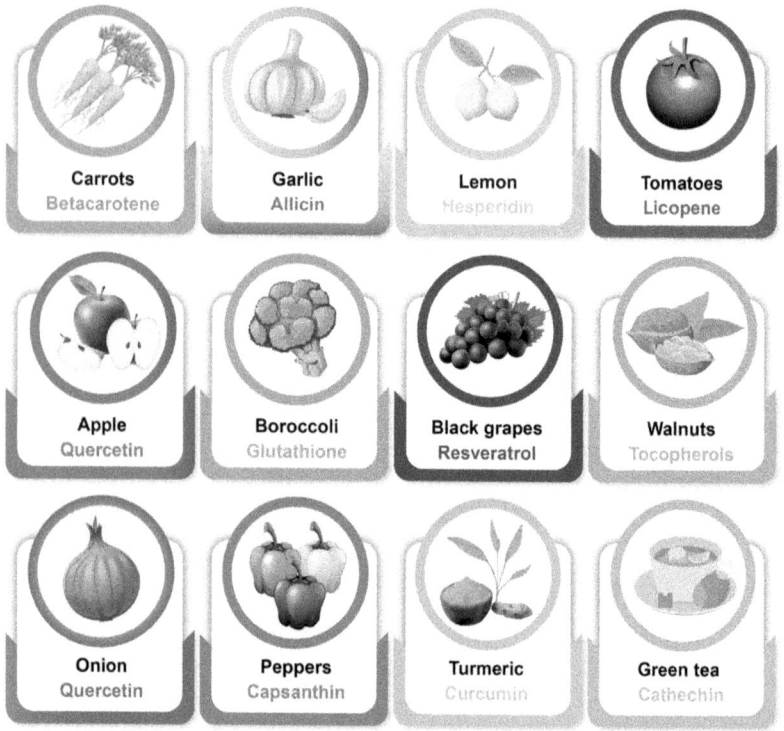

Figure 7: Antioxidants-rich diet.

You can get antioxidants from supplements, but Taylor recommends obtaining them from plant-based sources instead of those synthesised in a laboratory. Thus, she went on to infer that the basis of good nutrition, such as fruit, vegetables, nuts, seeds, and beans, hasn't changed, and if you're consuming animal protein, eat seafood and avoid processed meats.

There are several antioxidant-rich foods, but some are considered rich in antioxidants, as given below. The recommended daily values (DV) are available in the NIH Dietary Supplement Label Database:

I. **Blueberries:** They may be small but are highly nutritious. Blueberries are rich in vitamins and minerals and are also rich in anthocyanins with potent antioxidant properties. Blueberries are labeled superfoods for a reason and possess numerous health benefits, including enhancing brain function, promoting healthy and strong bones, and reducing the risk for heart disease [59]. A study published in May 2019 in The American Journal of Clinical Nutrition showed that eating a cup of blueberries daily for six months reduces the risk of heart disease by 12 to 15 percent.

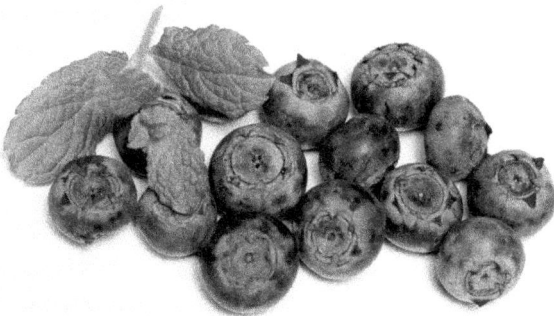

Here are the nutrition facts for 1 cup (148 g) of blueberries, according to the U.S. Department of Agriculture (USDA):

- Calories 84

- Protein 1.1 grams (g)

- Carbohydrates 21.5g

- Sugar 14.7g

- Fat 0.5g

- fibre 3.6g

- Calcium 9mg, or 1 percent of the DV

- Iron 0.4mg, or 3 percent of the DV

- Magnesium 9mg, or 2 percent of the DV

- Vitamin K 29mcg, or 24 percent of the DV

- Phosphorus 18mg, or 1 percent of the DV

- Vitamin A 80 IU, or 2 percent of the DV

- Potassium 114mg, or 2 percent of the DV

- Folate 9mcg, or 2 percent of the DV

- Vitamin C 14mg, or 16 percent of the DV

II. **Broccoli:** Like other dark and leafy vegetables, broccoli is rich in phenolics, which are essential for human health due to their high antioxidants and anti-cancer properties, which may protect against disease, inflammation, and allergies [60]

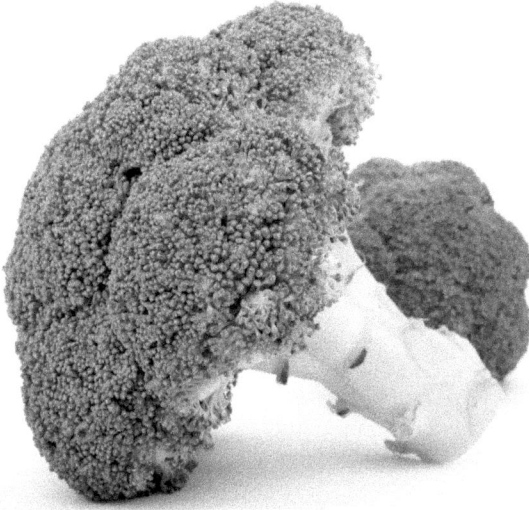

Here are the nutrition facts for 1 cup (91 g) of chopped broccoli, according to the USDA:

- Calories 31
- Protein 2.6g
- Fat 0.3g
- Carbohydrates 6g
- Sugar 1.6g
- Sodium 30mg

- Phosphorus 60mg, 5 percent of the DV

- Potassium 288mg, 6 percent of the DV

- Magnesium 19mg, or 5 percent of the DV

- fibre 2.4g

- Calcium 43mg, or 3 percent of the DV

- Iron 1mg, or 4 percent of the DV

- Vitamin C 81mg, or 90 percent of the DV

- Folate 57mcg, or 14 percent of the DV

- Vitamin A 567 IU, or 11 percent of the DV

- Vitamin K 93mcg, or 77 percent of the DV

III. **Walnuts:** They are rich in fibre, protein, and unsaturated fats and used in Chinese herbal medicine for brain health to help keep the brain cells healthy and improve memory, according to a study published in June 2016 in the journal Natural Product Communications. As confirmed by Harvard Health Publishing, walnuts are heart-healthy due to their polyunsaturated and monounsaturated fats. A review published in December 2017 in Nutrients cites that eating this Mediterranean diet in moderation may help you lose belly fat and reduce your risk for type 2 diabetes and heart disease. Walnuts have high polyphenol content with antioxidant properties to offset oxidative stress. They may help fight inflammation, promote weight control, and prevent diseases such as cancer, as cited in a study published in November 2017 in the Critical Reviews in Food Science and Nutrition.

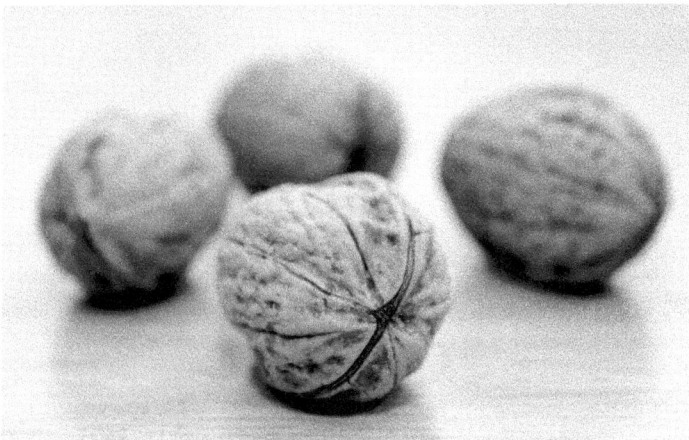

Here are the nutrition facts for ¼ cup (30 g) of walnuts, according to the USDA:

- Calories 200
- Protein 5g
- Fat 20g
- Sugar 1g
- Carbohydrates 4g
- fibre 2g
- Iron 1mg, or 4 percent of the DV
- Calcium 20mg, or 2 percent of the DV

IV. **Spinach**: A relative of the beetroot and a low-calorie vegetable loaded with nutrients that can promote eye, bone, and hair health. There is evidence linking lutein, a carotenoid in spinach that also gives carrots their orange hue, to promoting eye health and inhibiting age-related macular degeneration [47]. The antioxidant properties of lutein may also support heart health and reduce cancer risk.

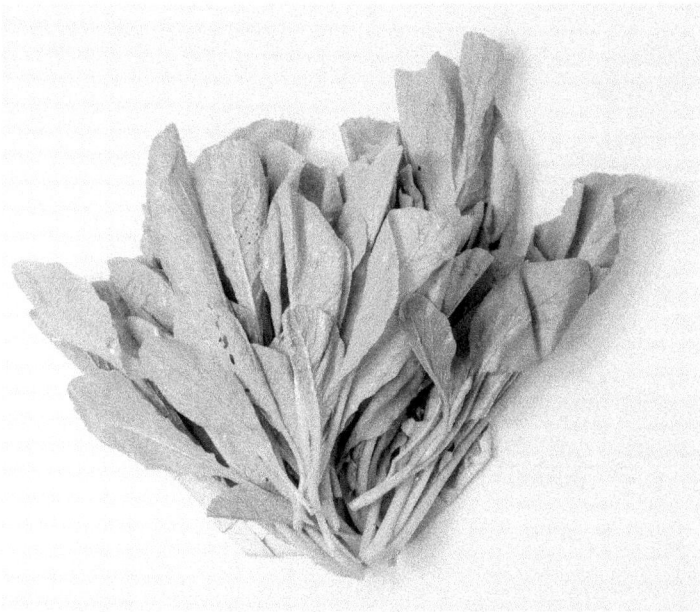

Here are the nutrition facts for 1 cup (30 g) of spinach, according to the USDA:

- Calories 7
- Protein 0.9g
- Carbohydrates 1.1g
- Fat 0.1g
- fibre 0.7g
- Sodium 24mg
- Sugar 0.1g
- Calcium 30mg, or 2 percent of the DV
- Iron 0.8mg, or 5 percent of the DV
- Phosphorus 15mg, or 13 percent of the DV
- Magnesium 24mg, or 6 percent of the DV
- Folate 58mcg, or 15 percent of the DV
- Potassium 167mg, or 4 percent of the DV
- Vitamin A 2813 IU, or 56 percent of the DV
- Vitamin C 8mg, or 9 percent of the DV
- Vitamin K 145mcg, or 121 percent of the DV

V. **Potatoes:** These tuberous vegetables are full of vitamins and minerals. To obtain the maximal health benefits, choose more colourful spuds, such as sweet or purple potatoes, for a higher concentration of antioxidants. Studies published in April 2016 in Critical Reviews in Food Science and Nutrition have discovered that potatoes' antioxidants may help reduce the risk of blood pressure, cancer, heart disease, and neurodegenerative diseases.

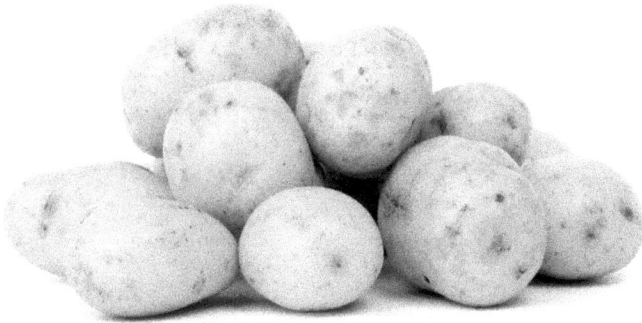

Here are the nutritional facts for one medium (213 g) russet potato (with skin), according to the USDA:

- Calories 168
- Fat 0.2g
- Protein 4.6g
- Sugar 1.3g
- Fibre 2.8g

- Carbohydrates 38.5g

- Iron 2mg, or 10 percent of the DV

- Calcium 28mg, or 2 percent of the DV

- Phosphorus 117mg, or 9 percent of the DV

- Magnesium 49mg, or 12 percent of the DV

- Zinc 1mg, or 6 percent of the DV

- Potassium 888mg, or 19 percent of the DV

- Vitamin C 12mg, or 13 percent of the DV

- Niacin 2mg, or 14 percent of the DV

- Folate 30mcg, or 8 percent of the DV

- Vitamin K 4mcg, or 3 percent of the DV

VI. **Green Tea:** Its rapid increase in popularity is due to its several health benefits, with research found anti-inflammatory, anticarcinogenic, and antimicrobial properties [61]. What differentiates green tea from other teas is the high number of catechins, a phytochemical that serves as a potent antioxidant. Catechins are popular antimicrobial agents, and studies, including the one cited, have discovered they can help treat and prevent infectious diseases [61].

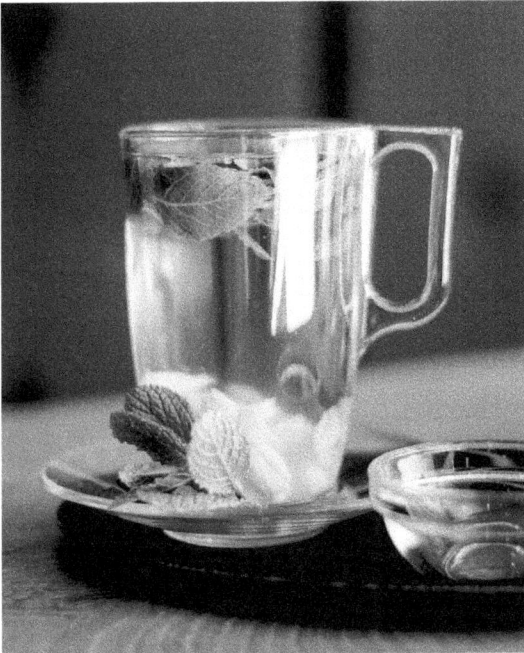

Here are the nutrition facts for 1 cup of brewed green tea (245 g), according to the USDA:

- Calories 2
- Protein 0.5g
- Riboflavin 0.1mg, or 11 percent of the DV

VII. **Strawberries:** Sweet and juicy strawberries are a pride of the berry family. Like blueberries, strawberries derive their specified red colour from anthocyanins, giving them their superfood status. Studies have found that strawberries may reduce inflammation and blood pressure, which could help prevent heart disease, according to a review published in July 2019 in the journal Nutrients. The polyphenols, the same compound in cranberries and spinach, may also enhance insulin sensitivity in overweight people without diabetes, which suggests it may help prevent type 2 diabetes, reported a study published in February 2017 in the British Journal of Nutrition.

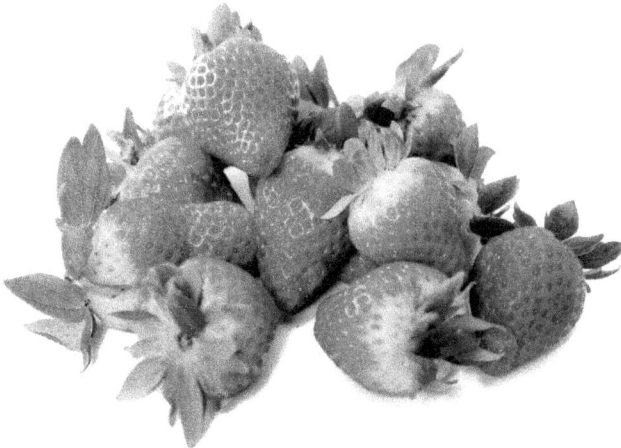

Here are the nutritional facts for 1 cup (152 g) of strawberry halves, according to the USDA:

- Calories 49
- Fibre 3.0g
- Carbohydrates 11.7g
- Protein 1.0g
- Fat 0.5g
- Sodium 2mg
- Sugar 7.4g
- Iron 1mg, or 3 percent of the DV
- Calcium 24mg, or 2 percent of the DV
- Phosphorus 36mg, or 3 percent of the DV
- Magnesium 20mg, or 5 percent of the DV
- Potassium 233mg, or 5 percent of the DV
- Niacin 0.6mg, or 4 percent of the DV
- Vitamin C 89mg, or 99 percent of the DV
- Vitamin E 0.4mg, or 3 percent of the DV
- Zinc 0.2mg, or 2 percent of the DV
- Folate 36mcg, or 9 percent of the DV
- Vitamin K 3mcg, or 3 percent of the DV

VIII. **Beans:** There are several types of edible beans, which are rich in fibre, phytochemicals, and protein. Beans are a staple in plant-based diets like vegetarian and vegan diets. According to a study published in November 2017 in the International Journal of Molecular Sciences, they contain nearly the same amount of protein as meat.

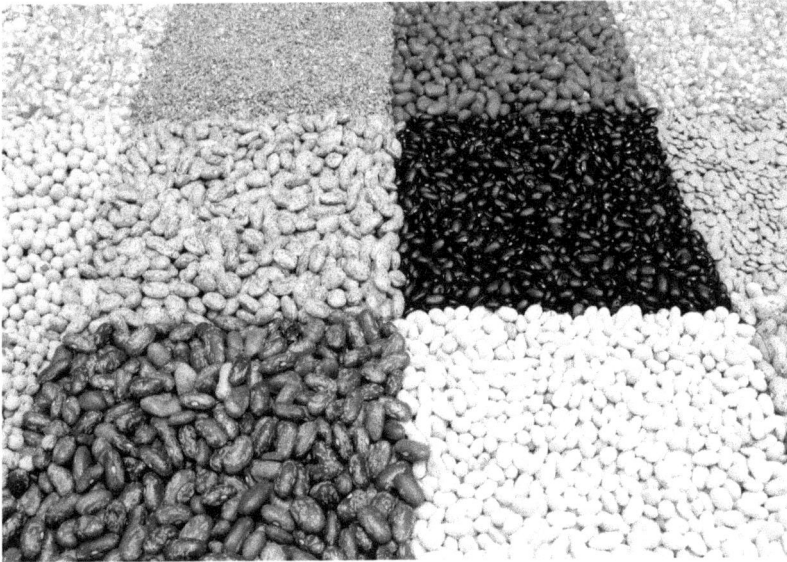

Here are the nutritional facts for 1 cup (266 g) of canned red kidney beans, drained and rinsed, according to the USDA:

- Calories 191
- Fat 1.5g
- Protein 12.8g

- Carbohydrates 32.9g

- Sodium 329mg

- fibre 9.5g

- Calcium 92mg, or 7 percent of the DV

- Magnesium 46mg, or 11 percent of the DV

- Iron 2mg, or 11 percent of the DV

- Phosphorus 186mg, or 15 percent of the DV

- Zinc 1mg, or 9 percent of the DV

- Folate 36mcg, or 9 percent of the DV

- Potassium 395mg, or 8 percent of the DV

- Thiamin 0.1mg, or 8 percent of the DV

- Niacin 1mg, or 8 percent of the DV

LIST OF ANTIOXIDANTS AND FOOD SOURCES:

There is evidence that antioxidants are more potent when taken from whole foods instead of isolated from a portion of food [31]. Various research studies have found that some vitamin supplements can increase your cancer risk. For instance, vitamin A (beta-carotene) consumption is linked with a reduced risk of certain cancers, while an increased risk of lung cancer in smokers is linked with purified vitamin A. Antioxidants are most abundant in fruits and vegetables, such as:

Catechins: Red wine and tea

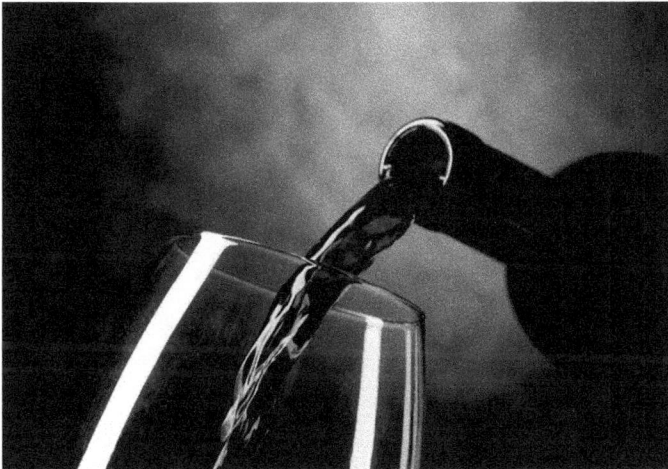

Allium sulphur compounds: Garlic, leeks, onions

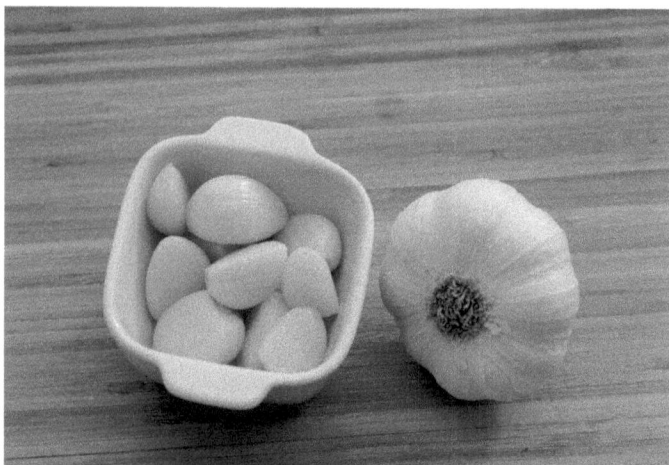

Beta-carotene: Pumpkin, carrots, spinach, mangoes, apricots, and parsley

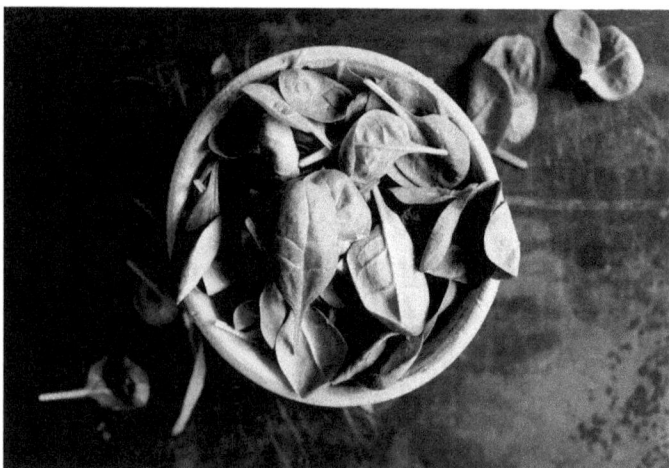

Anthocyanins: eggplant, grapes, and berries

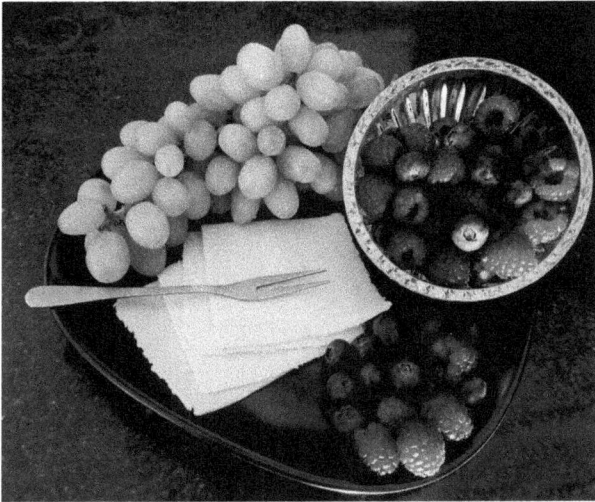

Copper: Seafood, milk, lean meat, and nuts

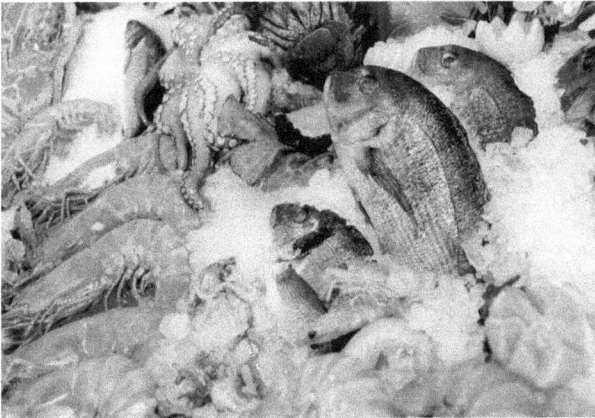

Flavonoids: red wine, tea, citrus fruits, green tea, onion, and apples

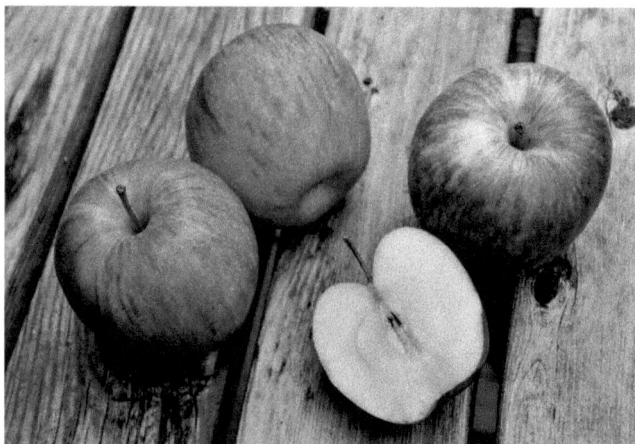

Cryptoxanthins: Pumpkin, red capsicum, and mangoes

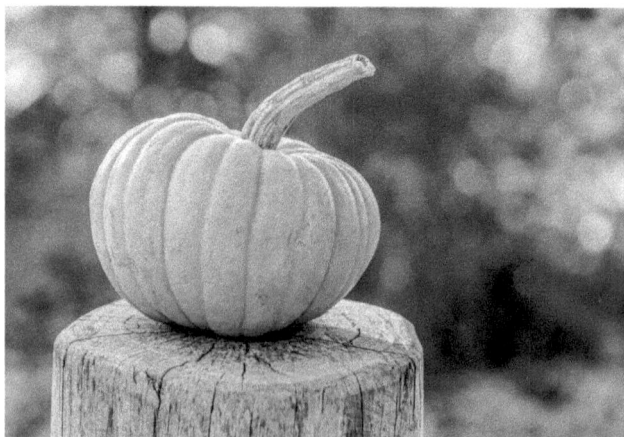

Lignans: whole grains, sesame seeds, bran, and vegetables

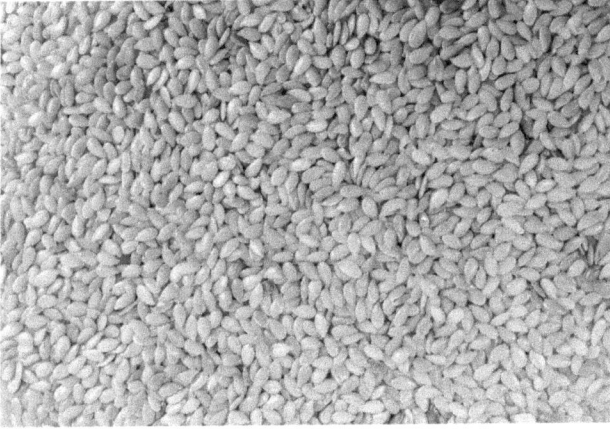

Indoles: Cruciferous vegetables, such as cabbage, broccoli, and cauliflower

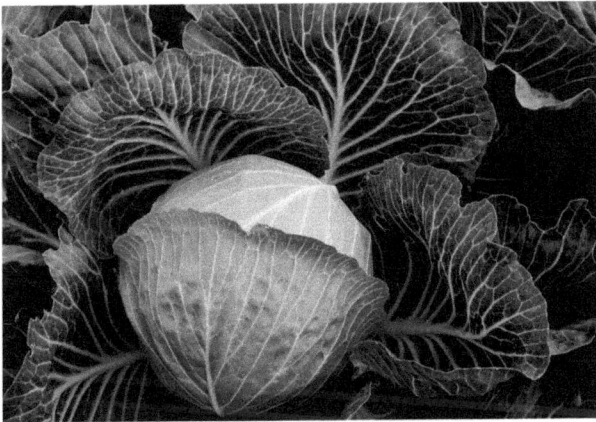

Lycopene: apricots, tomatoes, pink grapefruit, and watermelon

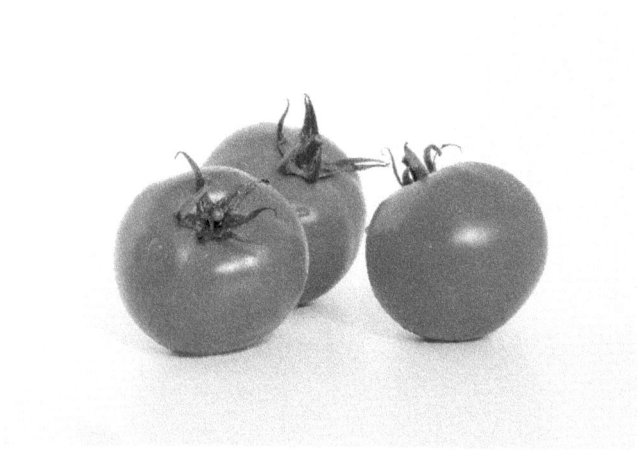

Isoflavonoids: tofu, soybeans, lentils, peas, and milk

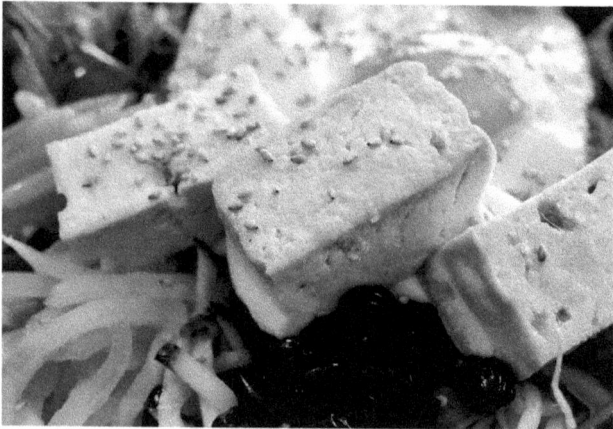

Lutein: Green and leafy vegetables like spinach, and corn

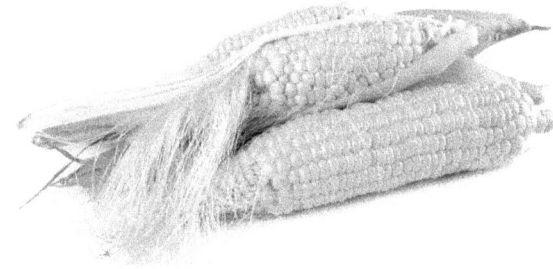

Manganese: lean meat, seafood, milk, and nuts

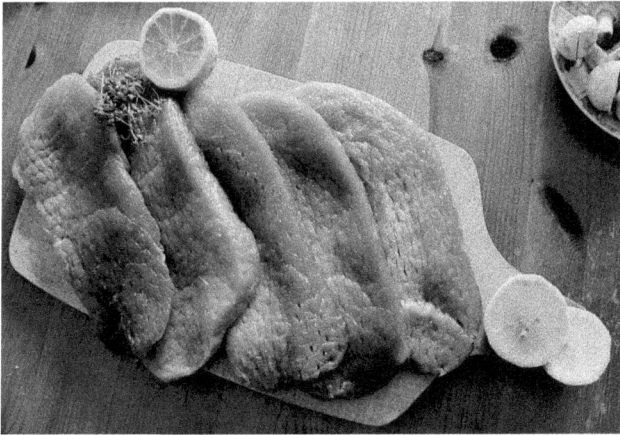

Polyphenols: Herbs

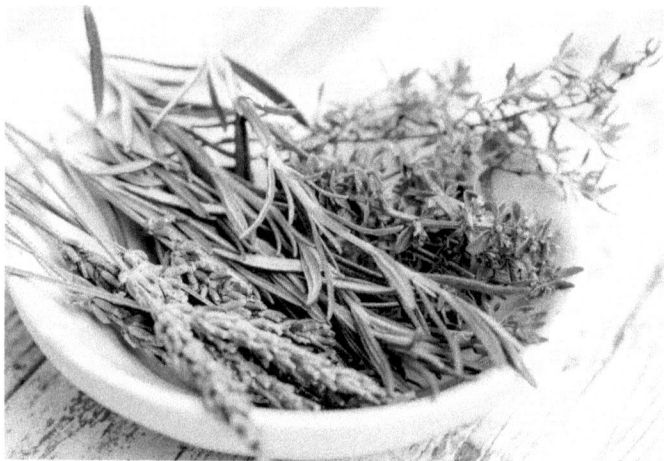

Vitamin A: Carrots, liver, sweet potatoes, milk, and egg yolks

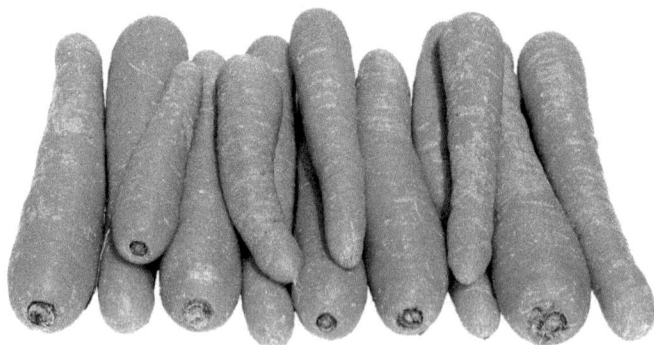

Selenium: Lean meat, seafood, offal, and whole grains

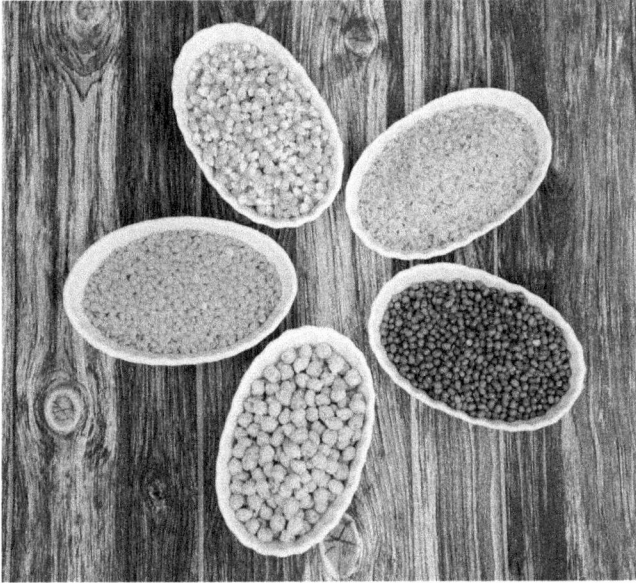

Vitamin C: Spinach, oranges, blackcurrants, mangoes, broccoli, kiwifruit, capsicum, and strawberries

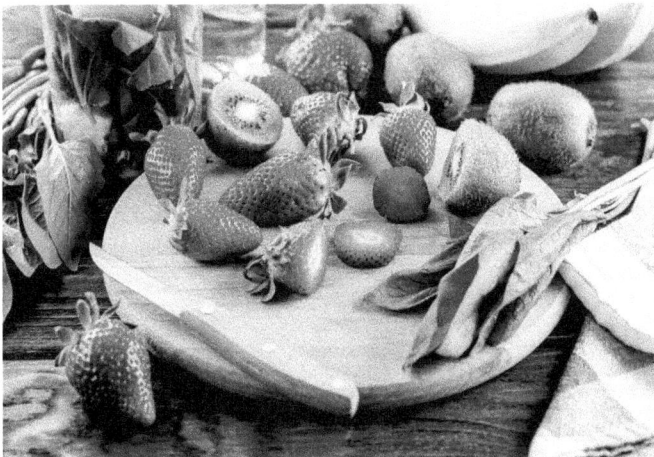

Zinc: Lean meat, seafood, milk, and nuts

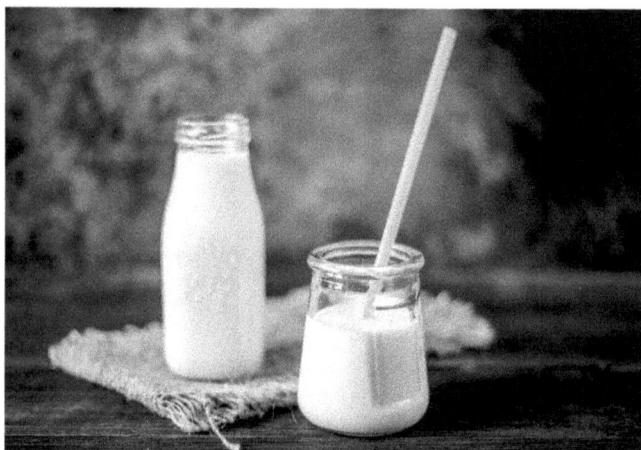

Vitamin E: Vegetable oils (such as wheatgerm oil), avocados, nuts, seeds, and whole grains

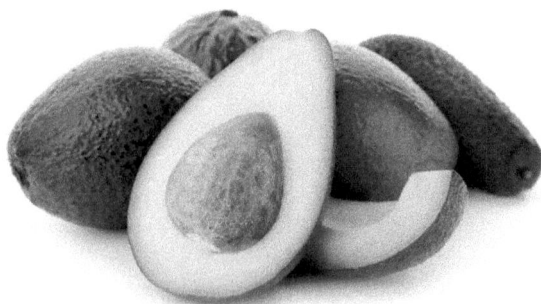

Zoochemicals: Offal, red meat, and fish. It can also be obtained from the plants that animals eat.

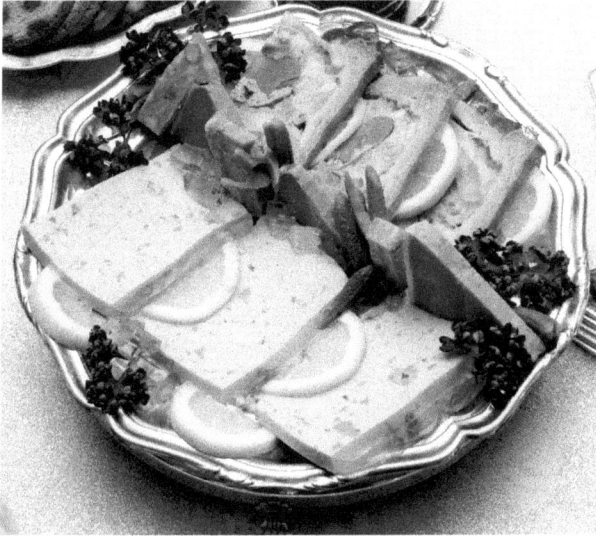

PART II:

CHAPTER FOUR

Molecular Basis of Ageing is the Shortening of DNA During Each Cycle of Replication

Ageing at the molecular and cellular levels is characterised by accumulative damage to cellular DNA, RNA, proteins, and other macromolecules [19]. Increased molecular heterogeneity is the fundamental basis for the cellular and physiological mutations that occur during ageing. The imperfections of the sustenance and repair systems that comprise the haemodynamic space contribute to a progressive failure of homeodynamics.

Telomerase is the enzyme responsible for maintaining an optimal length of the telomeres by adding guanine-rich repetitive sequences (figure 8). Higher telomerase activity is shown in gametes and stem and tumour cells. In human somatic cells, maturation potential is limited, and Senescence or cessation of cell division follows approximately 50-70 cell divisions [62]. On the other hand, the cellular replication capacity is nearly unlimited in most tumour cells. The critical role in maintaining telomere length with the engagement of telomerase is still inconclusive. DNA polymerase cannot fully copy DNA at the ends of chromosomes; therefore, about 50 nucleotides are lost during each cell cycle, resulting in a gradual telomere length shortening. Critically short telomeres engender Senescence and cell death. However, in tumour cells, the system of telomere length maintenance is stimulated. Apart from catalytic telomere elongation, independent telomerase functions can also be engaged in cell cycle regulation.

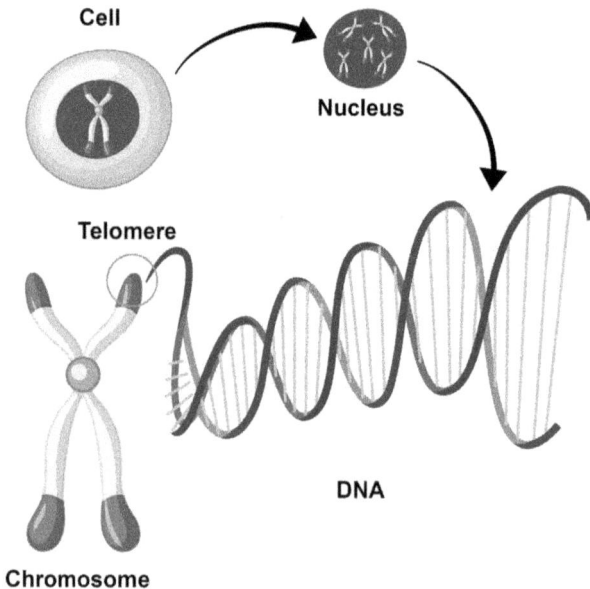

Figure 8: Telomere cap at the end of chromosomes protect DNA from damage during cell division.

Furthermore, the inhibition of telomerase catalytic function and the associated inability to maintain telomere length may help prevent tumour cell replication potential [63]. On the other hand, the formation of a temporarily active enzyme through its intracellular activation or due to stimulation of expression of telomerase components causes telomerase activation and telomere elongation that can be utilised for correction of degenerative changes [62]. Data on telomerase structure and function in this book are compared for remote evolutionary organisms. The problems of evaluating telomerase activity and its modulation by enzyme inhibitors or activators are also considered.

Every time your cells divide, the DNA in the new cells gets shorter. Primary age-related mutations include genomic instability, dysregulated gene expression, mutations, cellular Senescence, tissue disorganisation, elevated vulnerability to stress, impaired intercellular communication, organ dysfunctions, and reduced ability to adapt and remodel. Several approaches for intervention, prevention, and modulation of ageing target the occurrence and accumulation of molecular damage.

Mild stress-induced hormesis engendered by physical, biological, and nutritional hormesis is a promising and holistic strategy for strengthening cellular homeodynamics. Food components, which activate one or more pathways of stress response in cells and organisms, are nutritional hormetins and can possess some health- and longevity-promoting effects.

The evolutionary and biological basis of ageing is now well established, showing that any specific gerontogenes do not influence ageing. Instead, poor maintenance and compromised repair systems cause a progressive failure of homeodynamics, ageing, and eventual mortality. Several interventions for ageing, such as gene therapy, hormonal replenishment, stem cell therapy, and nutritional supplementations, experimented primarily on experimental model systems, have achieved limited human progress [64]. The complex trait of ageing requires holistic strategies for maintaining or improving health in old age. Therefore, a reliable health maintenance and improvement approach is "mild stress-induced physiological hormesis." Physical and mental exercise and several non-nutritional food components, such as polyphenols, flavonoids, and terpenoids in spices, oils, and other formulations, are hormetins, which possess health benefits by affecting physiological hormesis. The future expectation for ageing intervention and the molecular basis of ageing, as reflected in the shortening of DNA, include intelligent redesigning and trans-humanistic improvements through artificial intelligence and cyborgs combining organic and biomechatronic body parts.

TELOMERASE, LOCATION AND FUNCTION

Telomeres are a series of tens to thousands of nucleotides at the ends of chromosomes and are essential for stabilising the chromosomal ends and preventing breakage, translocation, and loss of DNA material [65]. During DNA replication, there is a progressive shortening of telomere length, which is the basis of cellular ageing and serves as a replicative senescence signal. In most cancers, telomerase□ encoded by theTERT gene, an enzyme that includes telomeres to the ends of chromosomes, becomes activated, usually via alterations in the TERT promoter [66]. The telomerase-driven telomere length maintenance in tumours facilitates unrestrained cellular maturation by relieving the central waypoint to cellular life span.

TELOMERASE IN SEX CELLS BUT NOT IN BODY CELLS:

Males and females usually age at different rates, which results in longevity 'gender gaps,' where one gender tends to outlive the other. Why the two genders have distinct lifespans is an age-old puzzle with no definite explanation. A cellular process related to lifespan, known to vary according to sex, is the rate at which the protective telomere chromosome caps are lost. Regarding humans, men have shorter lifespans and higher telomere shortening [66]. This has contributed to speculation by the scientific community that gender-based telomere shortening is one of the causes of gender-specific mortality. However, telomere shortening may be a cause for or a result of the processes that regulate survival. To project from a general viewpoint using single-taxon studies may be misleading. A review of recent work on telomeres utilizing a variety of animal taxa, including those with reverse sexual lifespan dimorphism, that is where males live longer, tried to establish whether sex-based survival is generally linked with sex differences in telomere dynamics.

TELOMERASE MODIFICATION TO PREVENT DNA SHORTENING AS A MEASURE TO IMPROVE LIFESPAN

Telomerase is a ribonucleoprotein complex that catalyses the inclusion of a telemoric sequence to the ends of chromosomes [65]. The catalytic protein component of telomerase is only expressed in specific germ line cells, maturation stem cells of renewal tissues, and cancer cells. The expression of hTERT (Telomerace Reverse Transcriptase) in typical cell reconstitutes telomerase activity and circumvents the induction of Senescence [65]. Telomere length regulation and maintenance contribute to typical human cellular ageing and diseases. The synthesis of telomeres is primarily regulated by the cellular reverse transcriptase telomerase, an RNA-dependent DNA polymerase that adds telomeric DNA to telomeres. Telomerase expression is usually needed for cell immortalisation and long-term tumour growth. In humans, telomerase activity is comprehensively regulated during development and oncogenesis. The regulation of telomerase activity may have important implications in anti-ageing and anti-cancer therapy.

The expression of hTERT in normal cells restructures telomerase activity and evades the induction of Senescence. Telomeres shorten with each cell division, ultimately leading to Senescence (ageing) due to incomplete lagging DNA strand synthesis and end-processing events and because telomerase activity is not observed in most somatic tissues [66]. There are specific tissues and areas where replicative Senescence participates in the decline in human physiological function with increased age and chronic illnesses. While expressing hTERT in cells results in the maintenance of telomere length and greatly extended life span, blocking replicative ageing would be systematically predicted to increase the potential for tumour formation. However, there are many situations in which the transient rejuvenation of cells could be beneficial. Ectopic expression of hTERT can immortalise human skin keratinocytes, dermal fibroblasts, muscle satellite (stem), and vascular endothelial, myometrial, retinal-pigmented, and breast epithelial cells in cell culture studies. In addition, human bronchial, corneal, and skin cells expressing hTERT can be used to form organotypic (3D) cultures (bioengineered tissues) that express differentiation-specific proteins, demonstrating that hTERT by itself does not alter normal physiology. The production of hTERT-engineered tissues offers the possibility of producing tissues to treat various chronic diseases and age-related medical conditions due to telomere-based replicative Senescence.

The concept of telomere originated in the late 1930s. Using cytogenetic approaches, Muller and McClintock discovered that the ends of the cellular chromosome, unlike random DNA breaks, possess unique properties that protect them from end-to-end fusion. Due to the extensive research in the past several years, many people have attempted to engineer the highly conserved telomere structures at the ends of linear chromosomes. The primary aim of these studies is to extend the lifespan and prevent the shortening of their DNA during cell division.

The telomeres' DNA sequence typically comprises tandem GT-rich repeats (TTAGGG), in humans and other vertebrates, with a single-stranded 3'-end projection that extends. Electron microscopy has observed that the single-stranded 3'-end overhang encroaches upon the duplex telomeric DNA repeat range to form a D-loop and T-loop structure in vitro studies. Telomere binding proteins sustain and modulate this distinct structure. The telomere is involved in several crucial biological functions. It safeguards chromosomes from recombination, end-to-end fusion, and recognition as damaged DNA; provides an outlet for complete replication of chromosomes; contributes to the functional organisation of chromosomes within the nucleus; engages in the regulation of gene expression; and serves as a molecular clock that regulates the replicative capacity of human cells and their entry into Senescence. Thus, it is challenging to engineer telomeres into cells

Replication of chromosomal ends poses a particular problem for cells. Watson and Olovnikov hypothesised that DNA should be progressively lost from the ends of chromosomes with every cell division. This is partly because the typical DNA polymerase could not fully reproduce the three ' ends of the lagging strands of the linear molecule (the end replication problem). Compatible with this hypothesis, telomere shortening is observed with progressive cellular division in cell culture models in-vitro and also with advancing age in in-vivo [66]. Typical mammalian somatic cells proliferate an insufficient number of times in vitro, with the maximum number being called the Hayflick limit [67]. This shortening in typical human cells functions as a molecular clock that regulates the replicative history of cells.

At the Hayflick limit, one or more critically shortened telomeres accelerate a continual growth arrest called replicative senescence or mortality stage 1 (M1) [67]. Cells that evade replicative Senescence by inactivation of a critical cell cycle checkpoint gene such as p53 continue to divide and exhibit further telomere loss until they attain a second proliferative block, catastrophe, or mortality stage 2 (M2), illustrated by massive cell death incited by critically short and dysfunctional telomeres. Rare survivor cells breaking out from crisis can retain telomere length, in most cases by activation of telomerase, which drives to infinite proliferative capacity, i.e., cellular immortalisation.

Telomerase is an RNA-dependent DNA polymerase that synthesises telomeric DNA sequences and almost universally contributes to the molecular basis for unlimited proliferative ability [65]. Since it was first discovered in Tetrahymena thermophila in 1985, it has been found that telomerase activity is absent in most typical human somatic cells but present in over 90% of cancerous cells and in in-vitro-immortalised cells. Telomerase comprises two essential components: the functional RNA component (in humans called hTR or hTERC), which serves as a template for telomeric DNA synthesis, and the catalytic protein (hTERT) with reverse transcriptase activity. hTR is highly expressed in all tissues despite telomerase activity, with cancer cells mostly having the fivefold-higher expression of telomerase than normal human cells. In contrast, the expression (mRNA) of the human catalytic particle hTERT is computed at less than 1 to 5 copies for each cell and is closely related to the cellular telomerase activity. hTERT is generally suppressed in typical cells and upregulated in immortal cells, implying that hTERT is the primary determinant for enzyme activity.

EFFECTS OF ANTIOXIDANTS ON LIFESPAN

Study shows that most antioxidants do not prolong the lifespan. If some antioxidants do lengthen lifespan, it is primarily due to their other activities, such as anti-inflammatory, epigenetic or mitochondrial actions. Why is it that most antioxidants don't work? Antioxidants, when taken orally, cannot reach the cellular compartments in an optimal concentration where they are most required. Notwithstanding, studies in which animals are genetically enhanced to produce higher antioxidant enzymes (like catalase) do not live longer. Such antioxidant enzymes function more effectively than antioxidants (small molecules) taken orally, but they do not affect lifespan significantly. Even more confusingly, accumulating evidence shows that the nutralization of free radicals by antioxidants can have life-extension effects. These effects are seen in worms, flies, and in rodents, including rats and mice. For example, chronic administration of different antioxidants significantly increases the average life of laboratory rats and mice. These antioxidants include vitamin E, some plant-based phytochemicals, royal jelly, and some cellular antioxidant enzymes [53-57]. In addition to improved lifespan, a significant improvement in healthspan is also noted in these animals. For example, they show better cognitive abilities, and improved functions of kidneys and liver after administration of antioxidants [53, 56]. However, it must be noted that several other studies contradict these findings and any inference should be cautiously drawn [57].

How could this be? Free radicals can function as a benign threat sign, boosting the cell's defense mechanisms, including detoxification enzymes and repair proteins, protecting our cells against age-related damage. That's why exercise is healthy. After all, during exercise, you produce a lot of free radicals because your cells must work extra harder. These exercise-induced free radicals activate all varieties of repair and defense mechanisms in your cells so that the cells can effectively protect themselves against the next time you exercise.

In the meantime, these improved defense and repair mechanisms also protect you against ageing and ageing-related diseases. Apart from exercise, vegetables, fruits, and green tea are healthy. This food contains slightly toxic substances, which boost detoxification and repair enzymes, making your body better protected against damage.

Healthy food contains substances that possess epigenetic effects that decrease inflammation, improve gut microbiome, do not overstimulate your ageing pathways (like mTOR or insulin receptors), and improve mitochondrial activities. Antioxidants can prolong your lifespan with the help of their free radical neutralising effect and rich vitamins and minerals content.

Conclusion

Oxidative stress in biological systems is a complex process characterised by an imbalance between the production of free radicals and the cellular ability to eradicate these reactive species with the help of endogenous and exogenous antioxidants. During the metabolic processes, a considerable variation of reactions occurs, where the boosters are the reactive oxygen species (ROS), such as hydrogen peroxide (H_2O_2) and the superoxide radical anion ($O_2^{\bullet-}$), among others. A bodily system in the presence of an excess of ROS can introduce several pathologies, from cardiovascular diseases to cancer growth. Bodily systems have antioxidant agents to neutralize free radicals and minimize damage to cellular structures. The endogenous antioxidants are enzymes, such as superoxide dismutase (SOD), catalase (CAT), glutathione peroxidase, or non-enzymatic compounds, such as bilirubin and albumin. When a high concentration of ROS is observed in a cell, the endogenous antioxidant systems gradually fail, compromising the cellular structure and function. To compensate for this deficit of antioxidants, the body can use exogenous antioxidants replenished through food, nutritional supplements, or pharmaceuticals. Among the most critical exogenous antioxidants are phenolic compounds, carotenoids, vitamins C, and some minerals such as Selenium and zinc.

The current assumption is that we age because our DNA gets shorter or the integrity of our DNA becomes compromised as we age. Our protein production becomes less and less efficient as the instructional information becomes less and less accurate. Any nutrient that can conserve the integrity of DNA tends to add life to our years by retaining the integrity of our cells and allowing them to make proteins efficiently.

-- Prince N. Agbedanu

References:

1. Hellwig, M., *The Chemistry of Protein Oxidation in Food.* Angew Chem Int Ed Engl, 2019. **58**(47): p. 16742-16763.

2. Bao, Y., et al., *Freezing of meat and aquatic food: Underlying mechanisms and implications on protein oxidation.* Compr Rev Food Sci Food Saf, 2021. **20**(6): p. 5548-5569.

3. Hellwig, M., *Analysis of Protein Oxidation in Food and Feed Products.* J Agric Food Chem, 2020. **68**(46): p. 12870-12885.

4. Slimen, I.B., et al., *Reactive oxygen species, heat stress and oxidative-induced mitochondrial damage.* A review. Int J Hyperthermia, 2014. **30**(7): p. 513-23.

5. Engwa, G.A., F.N. EnNwekegwa, and B.N. Nkeh-Chungag, *Free Radicals, Oxidative Stress-Related Diseases and Antioxidant Supplementation.* Altern Ther Health Med, 2022. **28**(1): p. 114-128.

6. Sadiq, I.Z., *Free radicals and oxidative stress: signaling mechanisms, redox basis for human diseases, and cell cycle regulation.* Curr Mol Med, 2021.

7. Scheibmeir, H.D., et al., *A review of free radicals and antioxidants for critical care nurses.* Intensive Crit Care Nurs, 2005. **21**(1): p. 24-8.

8. Nawaz, A., et al., *Protein oxidation in muscle-based products: Effects on physicochemical properties, quality concerns, and challenges to food industry.* Food Res Int, 2022. **157**: p. 111322.

9. Chanadang, S., K. Koppel, and G. Aldrich, *The Impact of Rendered Protein Meal Oxidation Level on Shelf-Life, Sensory Characteristics, and Acceptability in Extruded Pet Food.* Animals (Basel), 2016. **6**(8).

10. Soglia, F., M. Petracci, and P. Ertbjerg, *Novel DNPH-based method for determination of protein carbonylation in muscle and meat.* Food Chem, 2016. **197**(Pt A): p. 670-5.

11. Phaniendra, A., D.B. Jestadi, and L. Periyasamy, *Free radicals: properties, sources, targets, and their implication in various diseases.* Indian J Clin Biochem, 2015. **30**(1): p. 11-26.

12. Abrescia, P. and P. Golino, *Free radicals and antioxidants in cardiovascular diseases.* Expert Rev Cardiovasc Ther, 2005. **3**(1): p. 159-71.

13. Tamay-Cach, F., et al., *A review of the impact of oxidative stress and some antioxidant therapies on renal damage.* Ren Fail, 2016. **38**(2): p. 171-5.

14. Pizzino, G., et al., *Oxidative Stress: Harms and Benefits for Human Health.* Oxid Med Cell Longev, 2017. **2017**: p. 8416763.

15. Halliwell, B., *Role of free radicals in the neurodegenerative diseases: therapeutic implications for antioxidant treatment.* Drugs Aging, 2001. **18**(9): p. 685-716.

16. Huang, H. and K.G. Manton, *The role of oxidative damage in mitochondria during aging: a review.* Front Biosci, 2004. **9**: p. 1100-17.

17. Muriel, P., *Role of free radicals in liver diseases.* Hepatol Int, 2009. **3**(4): p. 526-36.

18. Nakai, K. and D. Tsuruta, *What Are Reactive Oxygen Species, Free Radicals, and Oxidative Stress in Skin Diseases?* Int J Mol Sci, 2021. **22**(19).

19. Kirkwood, T.B. and A. Kowald, *The free-radical theory of ageing--older, wiser and still alive: modelling positional effects of the primary targets of ROS reveals new support.* Bioessays, 2012. **34**(8): p. 692-700.

20. Yamazaki, I., H.S. Mason, and L. Piette, *Identification, by electron paramagnetic resonance spectroscopy, of free radicals generated from substrates by peroxidase.* J Biol Chem, 1960. **235**: p. 2444-9.

21. McCord, J.M. and I. Fridovich, *Superoxide dismutase. An enzymic function for erythrocuprein (hemocuprein).* J Biol Chem, 1969. **244**(22): p. 6049-55.

22. Dong, C., et al., *A comprehensive review on reactive oxygen species (ROS) in advanced oxidation processes (AOPs).* Chemosphere, 2022. **308**(Pt 1): p. 136205.

23. Mittal, C.K. and F. Murad, *Activation of guanylate cyclase by superoxide dismutase and hydroxyl radical: a physiological regulator of guanosine 3',5'-monophosphate formation.* Proc Natl Acad Sci U S A, 1977. **74**(10): p. 4360-4.

24. Halliwell, B., *Free radicals, reactive oxygen species and human disease: a critical evaluation with special reference to atherosclerosis.* Br J Exp Pathol, 1989. **70**(6): p. 737-57.

25. Sharma, G.N., G. Gupta, and P. Sharma, *A Comprehensive Review of Free Radicals, Antioxidants, and Their Relationship with Human Ailments.* Crit Rev Eukaryot Gene Expr, 2018. **28**(2): p. 139-154.

26. Blokhina, O., E. Virolainen, and K.V. Fagerstedt, *Antioxidants, oxidative damage and oxygen deprivation stress: a review.* Ann Bot, 2003. **91 Spec No:** p. 179-94.

27. Labat-Robert, J. and L. Robert, *Longevity and aging. Role of free radicals and xanthine oxidase. A review.* Pathol Biol (Paris), 2014. **62**(2): p. 61-6.

28. Kollarova, M., et al., *ZDF fa/fa rats show increasing heterogeneity in main parameters during ageing as confirmed by biometrics, oxidative stress markers and MMP activity.* Exp Physiol, 2022.

29. Poprac, P., et al., *Targeting Free Radicals in Oxidative Stress-Related Human Diseases.* Trends Pharmacol Sci, 2017. **38**(7): p. 592-607.

30. Avila-Nava, A., et al., *Oxalate Content and Antioxidant Activity of Different Ethnic Foods.* J Ren Nutr, 2021. **31**(1): p. 73-79.

31. Medina-Vera, I., et al., *Dietary Strategies by Foods with Antioxidant Effect on Nutritional Management of Dyslipidemias: A Systematic Review.* Antioxidants (Basel), 2021. **10**(2).

32. Konstantinidou, F., et al., *Impact of Cigarette Smoking on the Expression of Oxidative Stress-Related Genes in Cumulus Cells Retrieved from Healthy Women Undergoing IVF.* Int J Mol Sci, 2021. **22**(23).

33. Thirupathi, A., et al., *Effect of Running Exercise on Oxidative Stress Biomarkers: A Systematic Review.* Front Physiol, 2020. **11**: p. 610112.

34. Birlouez-Aragon, I. and F.J. Tessier, *Antioxidant vitamins and degenerative pathologies. A review of vitamin C.* J Nutr Health Aging, 2003. **7**(2): p. 103-9.

35. Olza, J., et al., *Reported Dietary Intake and Food Sources of Zinc, Selenium, and Vitamins A, E and C in the Spanish Population: Findings from the ANIBES Study.* Nutrients, 2017. **9**(7).

36. Coerdt, K.M., C.A. Goggins, and A. Khachemoune, *Vitamins A, B, C, and D: A Short Review for the Dermatologist.* Altern Ther Health Med, 2021. **27**(4): p. 41-49.

37. Asplund, K., *Antioxidant vitamins in the prevention of cardiovascular disease: a systematic review.* J Intern Med, 2002. **251**(5): p. 372-92.

38. Torre, M.F., et al., *Supplementation with Vitamins C and E and Exercise-Induced Delayed-Onset Muscle Soreness: A Systematic Review.* Antioxidants (Basel), 2021. **10**(2).

39. Al-Hashem, F.H., *Role of vitamins E and C in mitigating hypoxia- and exhaustive exercise-induced aberrant stem cell*

factor expression and impaired reproductive function in male *Wistar rats.* Saudi Med J, 2013. **34**(4): p. 354-63.

40. Canter, P.H., B. Wider, and E. Ernst, *The antioxidant vitamins A, C, E and selenium in the treatment of arthritis: a systematic review of randomized clinical trials.* Rheumatology (Oxford), 2007. **46**(8): p. 1223-33.

41. Taheri, S., et al., *A literature review on beneficial role of vitamins and trace elements: Evidence from published clinical studies.* J Trace Elem Med Biol, 2021. **67**: p. 126789.

42. Righi, F., et al., *Plant Feed Additives as Natural Alternatives to the Use of Synthetic Antioxidant Vitamins on Poultry Performances, Health, and Oxidative Status: A Review of the Literature in the Last 20 Years.* Antioxidants (Basel), 2021. **10**(5).

43. Saikiran, G., et al., *Selenium, oxidative stress and inflammatory markers in handicraft workers occupationally exposed to lead.* Arch Environ Occup Health, 2022. **77**(7): p. 561-567.

44. Gad, S.S., et al., *Selenium and silver nanoparticles: A new approach for treatment of bacterial and viral hepatic infections via modulating oxidative stress and DNA fragmentation.* J Biochem Mol Toxicol, 2022. **36**(3): p. e22972.

45. Alkadi, H., *A Review on Free Radicals and Antioxidants.* Infect Disord Drug Targets, 2020. **20**(1): p. 16-26.

46. Gong, Z., et al., *Associations Between Polymorphisms in Genes Related to Oxidative Stress and DNA Repair, Interactions With Serum Antioxidants, and Prostate Cancer Risk: Results From the Prostate Cancer Prevention Trial.* Front Oncol, 2021. **11**: p. 808715.

47. Mitra, S., et al., *Potential health benefits of carotenoid lutein: An updated review.* Food Chem Toxicol, 2021. **154**: p. 112328.

48. Hilton, J.W., *Antioxidants: function, types and necessity of inclusion in pet foods.* Can Vet J, 1989. **30**(8): p. 682-4.

49. Li, J., et al., *Evaluation and Monitoring of Superoxide Dismutase (SOD) Activity and its Clinical Significance in Gastric Cancer: A Systematic Review and Meta-Analysis.* Med Sci Monit, 2019. **25**: p. 2032-2042.

50. Zhang, Y., et al., *Association of total oxidant status, total antioxidant status, and malondialdehyde and catalase levels with psoriasis: a systematic review and meta-analysis.* Clin Rheumatol, 2019. **38**(10): p. 2659-2671.

51. Zinellu, A. and A.A. Mangoni, *A Systematic Review and Meta-Analysis of the Effect of Statins on Glutathione Peroxidase, Superoxide Dismutase, and Catalase.* Antioxidants (Basel), 2021. **10**(11).

52. Canals-Garzon, C., et al., *Effect of Antioxidant Supplementation on Markers of Oxidative Stress and Muscle Damage after Strength Exercise: A Systematic Review.* Int J Environ Res Public Health, 2022. **19**(3).

53. Quick, K.L., et al., *A carboxyfullerene SOD mimetic improves cognition and extends the lifespan of mice.* Neurobiol Aging, 2008. **29**(1): p. 117-28.

54. Inoue, S., et al., *Royal Jelly prolongs the life span of C3H/HeJ mice: correlation with reduced DNA damage.* Exp Gerontol, 2003. **38**(9): p. 965-9.

55. Anisimov, V.N., et al., *Effects of the mitochondria-targeted antioxidant SkQ1 on lifespan of rodents.* Aging (Albany NY), 2011. **3**(11): p. 1110-9.

56. Niu, Y., et al., *The phytochemical, EGCG, extends lifespan by reducing liver and kidney function damage and improving age-associated inflammation and oxidative stress in healthy rats.* Aging Cell, 2013. **12**(6): p. 1041-9.

57. Banks, R., J.R. Speakman, and C. Selman, *Vitamin E supplementation and mammalian lifespan*. Mol Nutr Food Res, 2010. **54**(5): p. 719-25.

58. Maciel, L.G., G.L. Teixeira, and J.M. Block, *Dataset on the phytochemicals, antioxidants, and minerals contents of pecan nut cake extracts obtained by ultrasound-assisted extraction coupled to a simplex-centroid design*. Data Brief, 2020. **28**: p. 105095.

59. Borges, G., et al., *Identification of flavonoid and phenolic antioxidants in black currants, blueberries, raspberries, red currants, and cranberries*. J Agric Food Chem, 2010. **58**(7): p. 3901-9.

60. Rodriguez-Hernandez Mdel, C., et al., *Natural antioxidants in purple sprouting broccoli under Mediterranean climate*. J Food Sci, 2012. **77**(10): p. C1058-63.

61. Vyas, T., et al., *Therapeutic effects of green tea as an antioxidant on oral health- A review*. J Family Med Prim Care, 2021. **10**(11): p. 3998-4001.

62. Tuttle, C.S.L., et al., *Senescence in tissue samples of humans with age-related diseases: A systematic review*. Ageing Res Rev, 2021. **68**: p. 101334.

63. Fakhri, S., et al., *Targeting cellular senescence in cancer by plant secondary metabolites: A systematic review.* Pharmacol Res, 2022. **177**: p. 105961.

64. Ohsawa, M., Y. Uezono, and A. Inui, *Editorial: Ageing-Related Symptoms, Kampo Medicine, and Treatment.* Front Nutr, 2021. **8**: p. 749320.

65. Shawi, M. and C. Autexier, Telomerase, senescence and ageing. Mech Ageing Dev, 2008. 129(1-2): p. 3-10.

66. Saretzki, G., Telomeres, *Telomerase and Ageing.* Subcell Biochem, 2018. **90**: p. 221-308.

67. Luft, F.C., *Approaching the Hayflick limit.* Trends Cardiovasc Med, 2015. **25**(3): p. 240-2.